Praise for Jessie's method

'Jessie has a gift to help you see the person you want to become.'

Avril, Dublin

'I was overweight and classed as obese for my height, weight, age. Pavelka Health taught me to keep going, one small step at a time, and this made something click in my head. I told myself, no more, this is a new start, a new chapter! I went to the gym and focused on me, and I fell in love with the feeling I got with exercise. I set myself challenges and goals, and with the support of the Pavelka Health Revolution family I am sure I will achieve them. My confidence is slowly building, as I can see the results from the hard work. How can I thank you again for changing my path in life? It's not about quick fixes it's about lifestyle, that's why Pavelka works!'

Ash, Wakefield

'For the first time ever, I am in control of what I eat, food does not control me.'

Margaret, Republic of Ireland

'I have a new-found love of exercise and the outdoors and have completed a 5K and climbed Mount Snowdon – both things I would never have believed I could do. My health has improved so much, including a marked decrease in the number of migraines I suffer. I feel more focused, living life "in the moment", concentrating on the things I can affect now, rather than worrying so much about yesterday or tomorrow, and making positive choices. It's a very a freeing experience.'

Emma, Somerset

'Jessie and Pavelka Health Revolution have motivated me to lose six stone and I have gained a zest for life I didn't know existed.'

Sharon, Cheshire

JESSIE PAVELKA

THE

PROGRAMME

for a leaner, stronger, healthier you

piatkus

PIATKUS

First published in the US in 2016 by Hachette Book Group, Inc.
First published in Great Britain in 2016 by Piatkus
1 3 5 7 9 10 8 6 4 2

A CIP catalogue record for this book is available from the British Library.

ISBN 978-0-349-41095-1

An imprint of
Little, Brown Book Group
Carmelite House
50 Victoria Embankment
London EC4Y 0DZ

An Hachette UK Company
www.hachette.co.uk

www.improvementzone.co.uk

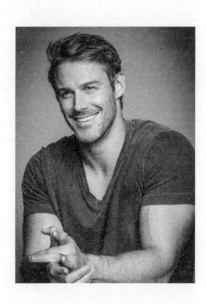

About the author

Jessie Pavelka is an internationally recognised fitness and well-being expert and specialist in extreme weight loss. He has worked on NBC's *The Biggest Loser*, as well as appearing on British screens with his life-changing work on *Obese: A Year to Save My Life* and *Fat: The Fight of My Life*. He's motivated the masses on Oprah's OWN Wake-up Workout, ITV's Motivation Nation in 2014 and headed the 'Sugar Free' campaign on *Good Morning Britain* in January and June 2015. Jessie is an ambassador for Cancer Research UK Race for Life, and has his own brand 'Pavelka', which offers a range of seminars, bootcamps and an interactive online community based around his philosophy of true health.

www.pavelka.co.uk

The Programme is dedicated to everyone who decides to take that first step towards something greater.
You'll never know how many lives you are changing.

Contents

Introduction:
How The Programme
Can Help You

··

My work as a trainer gives me the privilege of helping people take charge of their bodies and their lives. It is powerful to witness overweight and unhappy clients become confident, fit people. But losing weight is just part of the story: I have realised that true fitness is more than just physical. It is a gift to see the impact of fitness not only on the individual, but also on the people who love and care about them. I'm moved when I run into formerly sedentary clients with their children in the park, and see them climbing the jungle gym or on bike rides together. People who commit to improving their health don't only get in better physical shape: they often become more optimistic and engaged partners, parents and friends. They're inspiring. They're game. They're fun. Most of us are just plain happier when we're healthy. And when you're happier it's easier to make healthy choices and take care of yourself. The amazing part is that anyone can make profound and dramatic improvements in their lives by taking a few small steps, over and over. You need to move more, eat well, be mindful and connect with others. That's it, that's everything, and this book is going to show you how to do it right.

Over the years I've trained many people, with a diverse range of goals. Some clients are already pretty fit and looking to take things to the next level or to train for a specific sport or event. Others simply want to look their best for a school reunion. Other clients have been starting from tough places, maybe recovering from injury or illness, or have a significant amount of weight to lose in order to get healthy. The Programme has been designed for people at different starting points, with an understanding that our journeys to fitness never really end. But we all need to set goals, and then work our way towards them. The experience will vary for each of us, and you'll find a number of different ways to measure your progress as you move through The Programme. Chapter 2 takes a closer look at planning your journey to fitness and staying motivated along the way: the key to success is to keep your mind focused on *why* you have chosen to take a healthier path: we all need a 'why'.

This book has your 'how' covered and it's going to be easier than you think. As you follow The Programme, you'll be focusing on four key elements of fitness:

- Eating nutritious, delicious food. You are going to eat whole foods that fuel your workouts, promote your health and make you feel good.

- Moving more. You're going to build your strength and endurance, improve your agility and flexibility, boost your metabolism and feel more comfortable in your body.

- Living mindfully. You are going to take a few minutes each day to breathe, relax, reflect and remind yourself of what you want and how much you already have.

- Connecting with people who care about you. You are going to cultivate some key relationships – including the one you have with yourself – that will help sustain and inspire you to be your best self.

These elements can be summed up in four simple words: Eat, Sweat, Think and Connect. When you do these things, your body will get faster and stronger than it is right now. You will sleep better at night and be energised and empowered as you move through your day. You are going to have more patience and compassion for the people around you. And yes, if you follow The Programme, you are going to look better. But, more importantly, you are going to feel good – and be happier. The best part is that you can use The Programme for the rest of your life.

HOW THE BOOK WORKS

Part 1 explores these four essential building blocks of fitness in more detail. The meal plans are organised to support your body on the path to fitness and make it easy for you to swap foods around in a way that works best for you. You may be stronger in one area of your fitness than another, and The Programme workouts accommodate that: I've provided three different levels of workouts. Your personal situation will determine which of the mindfulness practices make the most sense to incorporate into your day in the long term, but I'll ask you to try some different approaches over a few weeks to figure that out. I have come to believe that connecting with others and creating a supportive network of relationships that feed your soul is a critical part of living well and directly impacts your physical fitness. I also recognise that it is a lifelong process, and hope that the encouragement and tools offered in The Programme help you to begin, or strengthen, key relationships in your life. So The Programme can be used by anyone, at any fitness level, in an ongoing way.

If Part 1 is the 'what' and the 'why', Part 2 is the 'how'. It shows you exactly how the diet plan works and gives you recipes to take you through the 21 days of The Programme. There's plenty of variety and you won't get bored of eating the delicious recipes on pages 247–304.

Part 2 also takes you through The Programme workouts. The training schedule on page 142 gives you an overview of the 21 days. After this you'll find a workout for every day of The Programme (beginning with four fitness assessments to enable you to decide which level is right for you), with photographs and captions describing how to perform each movement.

You can repeat the 21-day cycle as often as you like: there are many ways to vary the recipes, and you will certainly find your fitness improves in one or more areas – so take your workouts up a level. And once you get into the rhythm of living mindfully and cultivating relationships your horizon will expand as you become healthier and happier. Get ready to Eat, Sweat, Think and Connect your way to fitness.

CHAPTER 1

Why I Created The Programme

··

Sports and exercise have defined and saved my life. I grew up in Texas and spent most of my childhood playing outdoors. Farms, fields, the beach: if it was outside, I was messing around in it, working up a sweat. I played football from the time I was four years old, and I enjoyed sports in general. As I got older and became serious about shaping my body for sport-specific performance in different seasons, I started spending more time in gyms and found myself learning a lot about training. I also found that people wanted to talk about this with me and be able to do what I was doing. Eventually I realised that I could make some money this way, and got professionally certified as a trainer when I was nineteen. I've worked with thousands of clients since then and figured out a thing or two about true fitness and how to get it. That's why I've created The Programme. The Programme will help you lose weight if you need to, but it's not a diet. The Programme is really a practical guide to living well that you can follow for ever to be the strongest, happiest, best version of yourself.

Much of what I know about getting healthy is informed and inspired by my work with clients who have been seriously over-weight. I've learned so much from their journeys. Sometimes I'm asked about how I found myself working so often with people who want to lose extreme amounts of weight. Here's what happened. I was living in California in my early twenties and developed a business called Fit for You with a friend and trainer named David Ryla. We created Fit for You to specialise in weight loss and work with bariatric patients who were pre-paring for, or recovering from, weight-loss surgery. Now, my first clients as a trainer in Texas were generally people I had met in my own gym, and most of them were not overweight. The majority of them were already pretty fit and just wanting to get in better shape for themselves or their spouses, put on a little bit of muscle, or hit a performance goal for a specific sport. I was instinctively knowledgeable about that and enjoyed helping people reach those goals. The training experience with the Fit For You clients was very different, but I took to it right away.

WE ALL NEED A WHY

Here's the thing: whenever someone is training, they need a 'why'. Why are you here today? What is your motivation? Did you sign up for a triathlon you want to complete in a personal record time? Do you want to look your best for a wedding on the horizon? Is your school reunion coming up? Want a six-pack? These are all fine goals to work towards, and I can help you get there. But the Fit For You clients were training because they wanted to live. Literally. Most of them were more than 45kg (7st) overweight and many had developed medical prob-lems because of it. Someone who is facing bariatric surgery has become so unhealthy that a doctor has told them they need to get fitter, one way or another, in order to keep breathing.

When a person comes into the gym knowing it's a do or die situation, they usually work out with a special intensity. While they generally have a long road ahead of them, they also tend to see improvements very quickly. It is an amazing feeling to watch that person increase from eight reps of an exercise to twelve reps or go from walking for 10 minutes to being able to run a mile without stopping. The pride someone experiences in that situation is as inspiring to me as the weight they are losing or the strength they are building. Helping people discover, or rediscover, confidence in their bodies and hope in their lives made me feel like I was not just doing work I enjoyed but work that had the potential to be genuinely meaningful.

In addition to getting a great sense of satisfaction from training very overweight people, I was also getting a practical education about issues specific to clients dealing with extreme weight loss. For example, being heavy can strengthen your bones and help you develop certain muscles, but moving extra weight is hard work and tough on the body. Therefore, my focus with very overweight people is always to protect their knees and feet. I understand where they are physically vulnerable and that if they get injured in particular ways they'll have to stop almost before they start. So I was getting an education in how to help people set reasonable goals and meet them safely.

I was also learning about other physical aspects of this level of transformation, like pain and loose skin, as well as the psychological challenges involved in changing entrenched behaviour patterns and family relationships. Keeping people motivated when they are stalled, or transitioning to a weight maintenance plan, was different for every client. It was challenging, stimulating, rewarding work. My experience with these clients is part of why movement is fundamental to The Programme. It's an aspect of fitness that is often missing from books about weight loss. Being active increases your metabolism, provides a range of critical health benefits immediately, even when your weight is not optimal, and keeps you motivated. The reality is that people are more likely to maintain a healthy weight when they exercise regularly, and it's much easier to stay active when you find ways of moving that you look forward to. I've drawn on everything I know about working out to help you develop a plan for movement that you enjoy and that is safe and appropriate for your level of fitness so that you can stick with it, adjust it as you get stronger, and use your increased fitness to find other activities that continue to inspire you.

MY OWN PROGRESS

Even though I have not personally struggled with my weight, I found myself connecting very personally with the Fit for You clients when they talked about the ways that they had been using food to deal with unhappy experiences and feelings. It reminded me of the unhealthy behaviours and strategies I have used in my own life, with a similar lack of consciousness, to avoid my own feelings. Listening to these clients helped me look at my own life differently. Learning how to deal constructively with the challenges we all face, and understanding the role that fitness plays in our happiness, is what it's all about.

I became a professional trainer while I was still in college. Those years were a time of transition for me, as they are for so many people. I had been admitted to the University of North Texas and was immediately given a place on their football team. But I had broken my shoulder blade a few years earlier and was experiencing some problems from that old injury. To cut a long story short, I had to quit the team. I had no idea what a big impact it would have on me to stop playing.

As a young man without football, I was lost. I didn't understand that I'd had a lifelong relationship with football, and had no idea how to deal with the sadness that would follow ending it. Sports had played a huge role for me, psychologically, as I was growing up. When I struggled with emotional things as a kid, such as my parents' divorce when I was nine, playing sports had allowed me to channel uncomfortable feelings of loss and powerlessness, even if I wasn't aware of that. The routines and demands of being a four-season student athlete had provided the daily structure for most of my life up to that point. All of a sudden, that outlet was gone. I found myself with a lot of time on my hands, and I didn't always make great choices about how to spend it.

Now, I could not have explained any of this to you – or to myself – at the time. And I didn't really try to talk about my feelings with anyone else. But I was struggling. I coped, in part, by doing what I knew best: working out. I was already a regular user of weights and I continued to go to the gym every day. Exercise kept me grounded and I started to focus more on bodybuilding. I got into power moves: dead lifts, bench press, power clean. These were all things I had done before, with goals for getting bigger, stronger and faster in particular ways for specific sports or games. But without a sport to train for, my goal in the gym just became to get bigger and stronger, period. There was no end in sight, no sense of 'Here is where I'm happy, here is where I stop.'

When I look back on that time, I know that even though I was fit and strong, I was working out in a way that became unhealthy. And I can see that I was also kind of grieving, although I didn't regret the decision to stop playing football. It was just that for the first time I had to deal with my life without letting a sport distract me, and I didn't know how to do that. My response was to focus on the outside part of me. In addition to connecting with people at the gym who shared my enthusiasm for exercise, I also joined a fraternity. I made good friends there and it replaced some of that team-like camaraderie I was used to, but without the stabilising factor of sport. I was working out hard, socialising intensely, and was often exhausted.

I was getting a lot of good feedback about how strong I was becoming. The owner of the gym I worked out in encouraged me to try a bodybuilding competition. My girlfriend at the time had already done one, so she offered to help me train for it. Always up for a challenge, I enjoyed the process of training for a competition and learning how people can use weights and exercise to precisely manipulate their muscles and body composition to control how they look. It was different from the way I had worked out before and it felt good to have a purpose driving my gym time again. But the competition itself, with the music and the posing trunks and choreography, felt very uncomfortable to me. I didn't like it and knew that even though I was placed second, I'd never do another one. I guess everything happens for a reason, though, because that one competition got me noticed by Ed Connors, who was based in California and owned Gold's Gym. Ed rang me after seeing that competition and said something like, 'You have a future in fitness or bodybuilding,' and offered me a job.

It did not take much convincing to get me to move from Texas to California. I knew that I needed a change. I was partying about as hard as I was training, which I sensed was not sustainable. And I was ready for new challenges. Over the next few years, I experimented with different training techniques and fitness activities with all types of people, connected with other professionals who shared my interests, started Fit for You and learned about running a small business, began exploring other aspects of health, including nutrition and mindfulness practices, and helped build a gym. I was also working out hard and starting to do features and covers in fitness industry magazines. I learned a lot about creating successful strategies for training different types of clients, developed an understanding of the fitness industry as a whole, and figured out the kinds of things that would help me maintain some balance in my own life and create a vision for my future. More recently, my wide-ranging experiences have led to me working as a trainer on *The Biggest Loser* and Sky TV's *Obese: A Year to Save My Life*. Both shows focus on the struggles of life when dealing with obesity. It enabled me to see the power of the human spirit and how small changes add up to real change and, in some cases, a miracle.

THE POWER OF EXERCISE

Exercise has been my anchor. When I go to the gym, life is just not that bad. Using my body helps to remind me that I'm alive and sometimes it allows emotion to move around and come to the front of my brain and release itself in unexpected ways. One of the things I've learned from my clients is how we carry emotions in different parts of our bodies and that exercise can allow us to release them. If you want to find a way to get to the core of a problem for someone, get them moving: when they are exhausted, all those filters they put in place to protect themselves fall away and you can figure out what is going on.

When people break down on *The Biggest Loser* or *Obese: A Year to Save My Life*, it's usually after they've been working out so hard their filters have dropped away. It's pretty incredible that that can happen through exercise, and it doesn't actually make you feel like something is wrong. As we grow up, many of us get the message that if we feel like crying, we should deal with it privately, that we shouldn't be feeling this way and certainly not showing it. But it's a good thing to know that it's OK for things not to be OK. And when they aren't, you might cry. Once you acknowledge whatever it is that isn't OK, you can start to deal with it. For many of the people I work with, gaining weight was a slow process of avoiding dealing with uncomfortable feelings.

MAKING CONNECTIONS

Listening to my clients changed my training methods. I began paying more attention to the mind–body connection, started understanding the difference between changing the body for health versus appearance and developed a deeper appreciation of the spiritual side of exercise. I came to realise how often we neglect this important aspect of fitness.

Often we start the day off strong, at full power, but as we move through it we have little interactions and experiences that drain us of our power and commitment: we run late, our kids give us a hard time, our boss is in a bad mood, we get bad news in the mail, something in the house breaks, stuff happens that distracts and depletes us, and, as a result, we make unhealthy choices without even thinking about it. The Programme incorporates different strategies to help you harness your mind power at the beginning and end of each day. You can use specific techniques at any moment to stay calm and centred, and remind yourself what is really important and how you want to live. These include writing in a journal, meditation and simple breathing techniques that are truly effective for staying committed to your best interests.

The Programme is going to teach you how to eat more mindfully, with an awareness of when and how to fuel your body for maximum performance and health. The mindfulness techniques I'll be asking you to try can benefit anyone, in a variety of ways, but they have been especially useful for my clients who have a history of eating or drinking in order to avoid feeling bad (or bored or frustrated). It's not a magic bullet, of course, but being intentionally conscious about what you feel, and when and why you want to eat, usually helps people make better choices about food. The mindfulness practices also help many of my clients realise how much better they feel when they move more.

Although I love the gym, there is also something special to me about exercising outdoors, and I'll be encouraging you to get outside during The Programme. Hiking is one of my favourite activities. It's great because you're moving, but there is also the possibility of a sense of connection to something greater than yourself. If you are moved by watching an amazing sunset, it might just be because it's beautiful, but I'd like to think there's something else going on there. It's a moment when you can say, 'Are my issues really that significant when I look at this sky?' For me, nature is both grounding and inspirational. I spent a lot of time at the beach with my family when I was growing up, and being outdoors near the Pacific Ocean is one of my favourite parts of living in California. There is probably a landscape that you find especially inspirational, and if there isn't, maybe you'll discover one as you begin moving and exploring more outside.

Wherever you wind up exercising, you may find that in addition to making you physically stronger, working out can be a time when you get very creative. I find that I can get a 'flow' going on a hike or at the gym that is almost meditative and that sometimes I can really sort things out in my mind. Working out reminds me that some things might be wrong but I still have this body. It also feels great: when I leave the gym after a hard workout, I am buzzing from the serotonin and dopamine my body releases. You don't have to understand the chemical process to know when you feel good, and I promise that you can't help but feel good when you give yourself the gift of movement and exercise. You'll also find that feeling good helps you make positive choices about the food you cook and eat.

Feeling good about yourself also makes it easier to have good relationships with other people who can support you on your journey and remind you of your purpose. Many of the people I work with who are trying to lose a lot of weight have really isolated themselves, and I understand that. It's hard to stay connected to others when you're feeling unhappy. But being isolated is one of the worst things you can do. I know that I make stronger, healthier decisions when I'm actively checking in with my family, especially my parents and my sisters. Being connected to people who care about you – not necessarily blood relatives – is a key part of The Programme. Don't be tempted to skip over that section if it doesn't seem like your relationships are directly related to fitness or weight loss. I have learned from my clients, and in my own life, that true fitness emanates from both inside and outside the body. Connecting with others helps you get there and stay there.

CHALLENGE YOURSELF TO CHANGE

Don't be alarmed if the idea of connecting with others to improve your fitness is a new one for you. It's important to step out of your comfort zone. Working on this book has been rewarding but also challenging for me: writing is a real change of lens in my world, where physical exercise has always been easy. It's OK – it's good! – if some aspects of The Programme are more challenging for you than others. We don't change without being challenged. And it's OK to be flat-out scared. One of my favourite things on some of the television shows I've worked on is to have people try a fitness activity that forces them to face some sort of personal anxiety. Sometimes it's water, sometimes it's heights: the exhilaration someone experiences after conquering their fear is contagious and inspiring. Often a person's fear is not so specific, but more a general kind of distrust about whether they can really get healthy and fit. I don't have to know anything about you to know that it's possible to improve your fitness, that how far you can go requires challenging yourself, and that your effort will be worth it. Once you decide you're going to do something, and you've done your homework so that you know it's safe, try to get out of your own way and just dive in and try it. Sometimes I tell people I work with 'Don't think too much, just jump off the cliff.' It's not the most gentle approach, and I guess it's my own version of feel the fear and do it anyway. But, really, once you make a decision, acknowledge the doubt and jump. Give yourself a chance to be surprised.

Maybe you have tried to lose weight before and it didn't go so well. Or maybe it went really well but you gained it all back. That's common. Almost any reasonable diet will work when you're following it, but most of them aren't realistic, or flexible enough, to stay on for the long term. Fundamentally, your weight is only one component of your fitness. If you can make a commitment to eat, sweat, think and connect with hope and intention every day, you're going to become more fit in every way that matters and probably be happier. You might even think about your weight loss as a kind of happy side effect of treating yourself well.

It takes conscious effort to make permanent changes to live well, and The Programme will show you how to do it. If you've picked up this book, you probably aren't exactly where you want to be right now. You might be scared to start or fail. It's OK. If this is you, I don't care how out of shape or unhappy you are, I promise that things are not as bad as they seem. You can make changes and it can happen right now. This may feel like jumping off a cliff, but you can start with some really simple steps. Get up and get moving. Believe in yourself and be hopeful. Focus on taking action that will make you feel good in your own skin today. You're not just going to chase a distant goal, although it's fine to set one. But if you take the actions I lay out in The Programme, you are going to feel better right now. And this all gets easier as time passes. The longer you stick with The Programme, the stronger you'll be.

Making healthy choices over the long haul gets easier because you develop good habits and self-discipline, but it also requires you to constantly renew your motivation. I'm a father now and it has changed my life in every imaginable way. My son, Rowan, causes me to look at so many aspects of life differently, from being more concerned about the quality of the food we eat and the environment we live in, to a renewed consciousness about the larger impact of my own actions and decisions. Rowan is only six and already I can see how fast our time together is moving. He makes me want to really be present and appreciate every moment we have together. Just hanging out with him, whether we're playing outside, building Lego or drawing, is an inspirational reminder of why I want to be the healthiest, strongest, best version of myself for as long as I possibly can.

Now it's time for you to think about your 'why'. Let's get started.

PART 1

The Key Elements of
THE PROGRAMME

CHAPTER 2

Setting Goals and Staying Motivated

FIGURE OUT YOUR WHY

One of the best parts of my job is seeing people reach their goals. The goals of the people I've worked with have varied tremendously. I've had clients who were essentially fit but wanted to get stronger or faster for an event or a race of some kind. Some clients are recovering from illness or injury. Some of my clients, at all different kinds of weights and fitness levels, have been miserable and depressed, and felt that being healthier would help them feel happier, find love, find more fulfilling work, or be better parents to their children. Other clients, although very overweight, had been quite satisfied and happy with their lives, but came to me when they were faced with a major health scare or crisis and they needed to get healthier in order to avoid a massive sacrifice in the quality of their lives. Some people's goals are very personal: I worked with a sweet woman who lived on a beautiful farm and had always loved horses, but she weighed 190kg (30st) and could no longer do much of anything.

She had limited mobility, was deeply depressed, and feeding and caring for her horses was just about the only form of physical activity she engaged in; the rest of the day was spent sitting on her sofa. Her goal was to be able to ride a horse again. So we burned that sofa – literally! – and set our goal to get her to a weight where she could safely ride a horse and start engaging in life again, and then take it from there. She reached her goal at 130kg (20st).

I don't know what your 'why' is, but one thing I've learned is that figuring out what it is, and keeping your 'why' in the forefront of your mind, is the key to living a healthy, well-balanced life. In the same way that our whys can vary, so can the ways we measure progress as we move towards our goals.

TRACKING YOUR PROGRESS

You need to set some goals. Let's say you want to lose weight. I don't know what you weigh now, what you want to weigh, and how long it will take you to get from here to there, based on your current fitness level. Here's what I do know: you can get there. You will enjoy the journey more than you think you're going to. It will probably be slower than you think it's going to be. It will be easier to keep faith with yourself if you track your progress. There are a number of ways to do that.

The scales

I'll be honest, I personally don't use scales. I know that might sound funny in light of my work on *The Biggest Loser* and I know many people find them to be a useful tool. So if that's you, go ahead and weigh yourself – but then put them away for two weeks. One week if you can't wait two. But, really, no more than that, because your weight will fluctuate from day to day for a bunch of different reasons and I don't want you to get demoralised over a number that reflects that you drank a lot of water. Weighing yourself once a week or every two weeks will be a more accurate reality check and be less apt to drive you crazy. Keep a few things in mind if this is how you are going to measure your progress: first, it will be most accurate if you weigh yourself under the same conditions each time you do it (at the same time of day and wearing the same type of clothing) and, second, if you are building more lean muscle mass, the scales may not reflect your real progress because muscle weighs more than fat. There may be times when you worked very hard for a week, really improved your mood and body in a variety of ways, and yet see a number on the scales that is disappointing to you. It can be a true test of character to push through that, but some people get discouraged by it, and there are other legitimate ways of assessing your progress.

Body measurements

It takes longer to measure parts of your body than it does to step on the scales, but this way of tracking changes can be very encouraging, since you will usually feel positive about one or more of the measurements even if another one is disappointing. You can measure your neck, chest, shoulders, arms, waist, hips, thighs and calves, using an ordinary soft tape measure. I recommend taking these no more than once every two weeks.

If you want to do this, be as precise as you can, but don't stress too much. As long as you keep your measuring methods consistent from week to week, you'll be tracking changes in your body accurately. For all the measurements, keep the tape measure parallel to the floor and flat on your body without pressing too hard.

Arms: Place the tape measure all the way around the widest part of your arm above the elbow (the middle of the biceps).

Calves: While you're standing up, place the tape measure around the widest point of your calves.

Hips: Place the tape measure around the widest point of your hips, right across your hip bones and buttocks.

Thighs: Place the tape measure around the widest point of your thigh.

Waist: Place the tape measure all the way around your torso around your natural waist, about an inch above your belly button. Don't suck in your stomach!

Chest: Place the tape measure all the way around the fullest part of your chest, across your nipples.

For some people, recording these six numbers every few weeks provides motivating feedback on their progress.

Clothes

Do you have a pair of jeans or a dress that you would like to fit into (or back into)? Try them on once a week and watch yourself get closer to your goal. You know this is a reality check because when your ordinary jeans start to feel tight is how many of us notice if we have gained weight. This works best if the item is fairly fitted as opposed to a loosely sized (small, medium, large) garment made from a stretchy fabric or with an elasticated waist. One thing to keep in mind: if your motivational clothing item is much smaller than you currently are, keep it to inspire you but consider getting something else you like, within two or three sizes of your current size, to use as an intermediate test of your progress. Some people find this to be a concrete and satisfying form of motivation and reward.

Body fat percentage

This requires going to a gym or a doctor or getting your hands on some equipment, because I'm guessing you don't have calipers or other instruments of body composition analysis in your house. But these tools exist, with varying degrees of accuracy, and you can have an assessment done, and then have it repeated on a regular basis. If this is something you want to do, make sure the follow-up uses the same method as the original measurement.

Exercise assessments

Pick a few – let's say four – exercises (you could use ones from the fitness assessments on The Programme, beginning on page 146) and record your progress every week. You could see how many press-ups, sit-ups or squat thrusts (burpees) you can do in 60 seconds, or time how long you can hold a plank or a wall sit. You can also time how long it takes you to walk or run a mile. Whichever exercises you choose, you can practise them as part of your workout routine and then do the timed tests once a week. These can be very motivating, because, like the body measurements, you'll almost always have an encouraging result in one area even if you are disappointed in another. It's also a nice way of reminding yourself how much stronger you are getting.

The feel-good scale

Are you a numbers person? Try looking beyond the number on the scales. There are four main elements to The Programme: I want you to Eat, Sweat, Think and Connect in a way that promotes your health every day. These will be described in full in the next four chapters. At the end of each day, consider whether and how you acted in each of these areas, and if you want to give yourself a score, try this:

- **Eat**: Did each of your main meals follow the recommended PCF (that's protein, carbohydrate and fat) ratio for the day (see page 62)? Give yourself 1 point for each meal that hit your target (total possible = 3 points)

- **Sweat** (see Chapter 4): Did you do both workouts today? Give yourself 1 point for each one you completed (total possible = 2 points)

- **Think** (see Chapter 5): Did you set an intention, take a moment to breathe, try a mindfulness activity and record three grateful or happy moments? Give yourself 1 point for each opportunity you took to be mindful (total possible = 4 points)

- **Connect** (see Chapter 6): I'll be asking you to work on four key relationships during The Programme but, unlike the mindfulness activities, most of this work takes more than a few minutes, so I don't expect you to do something in each area every day. Did you do one thing today to connect in a healthy way to yourself, a higher power, other people, or the wider world? Did you touch base with your accountability partner? Did you take a new class? Did you go for a bike ride with your children or a friend? Walk in nature? Call your mum or dad? Give yourself 1 point if you connected with someone (total possible = 1 point)

That's a somewhat arbitrary 10-point scale. Some people find themselves very motivated by a number, and if wanting that tenth point reminds you to take a moment to set an intention in the morning, that's great. If you score a 10, you'll be feeling like the day treated you pretty well, and it's because you took actions that encouraged that outcome. If you find you're consistently scoring lower, look at your patterns to see where you can try different strategies.

How do you feel?

This is a variation of the feel-good scale but without the point system. It is still an intentional assessment. Take some time each week to reflect on your progress. You can write this down if you like, but you don't have to. How did you do this week? Ask yourself all the same questions you would if you were using the feel-good scale, and consider what is working and not working, whether there is anything you can do to troubleshoot in the places that you're stumbling, and to reward yourself for what is going well. Think about how you are feeling. Are you happier? Calmer? More energised? Think about your 'why'. Do you feel like you're making progress towards that goal?

KEEPING A TRAINING JOURNAL

Some of my clients find it helpful to keep a record of their physical training. They take a couple of minutes each day to record the amount of time or distance they walked, or how many press-ups they did, or miles they biked, and note any unusual

▶

details about the workout. People who like doing this find it satisfying to review their progress and notice patterns over time to help them train more effectively. Other people find it stressful to keep track of their numbers in this way; it's definitely not for everyone. Try it if you think you might find it motivating; many people find it to be a powerful tool. If you decide to keep a training journal, I recommend keeping it as a separate file or notebook from your gratitude list (see page 121).

STAYING MOTIVATED

You are going to have moments when you don't want to exercise, even though you know it's good for you and you know you are going to feel better after you do it. Everyone needs motivation, even me sometimes. But I've found that if you take the body, the mind will follow. Tell yourself you can do 5 minutes. That's it, just put your trainers on, commit to 5 minutes, and do it. That 5 minutes will almost always turn into more and you'll be glad you did it. It's really that simple.

Sometimes I have clients who are very motivated to work out and are working hard, but reach a moment when they get discouraged because they hit a plateau in their weight loss. The reality is that the body adapts quickly and this is often a message that you need to do a little more. When I troubleshoot with people in this situation, making sure that they're clear and realistic about what they have been eating and how much they've been moving, often we'll find that something has gone off track. But when someone has truly been sticking to their plan and isn't seeing it translate into numbers on the scales, I try to help people look at this potentially frustrating time as a kind of gift. Even a moment for celebration. You are graduating to a new phase of your training, where you can take on more responsibility and push the boundaries of your potential. If you've been walking, maybe you're ready to run. That's an amazing moment.

The toughest moments are when it's just you, alone, surrounded by potentially bad choices with precarious motivation and no trainer to perform for, no fans in the stands, and no accountability partner. At those times you have to challenge yourself to be the best, most powerful version of yourself and remind yourself *why* you're doing this. Knowing that it's not all about the scales helps people stay motivated.

CHAPTER 3

EAT

....

Food is fuel. Athletes don't diet, they eat, and there is a direct correlation between nutrition and performance. The food that I'm recommending you eat on The Programme will help you meet your nutritional needs, maximise your performance when you work out, aid your digestion, and improve your health and your mood. If your diet is a fairly average one right now, you're going to lose weight over the next few weeks if you follow my plan. And you are definitely going to feel better.

Many weight-loss plans will tell you that a calorie is a calorie, no matter where it comes from. But the reality is that everything you eat affects your blood chemistry, and in the same way that you need to do the right type of training to get the most out of your workouts, you need to eat for high performance. Most, if not all, of the food you eat should be nutritionally dense and aimed at increasing your health and strength. This means that most processed foods, which have generally been stripped of their nutrients, vitamins and minerals, are no longer going to have a place in your cupboards and on your table. It's not only what's missing from these foods, but how your body processes them that's problematic: white flour and sugar increase the enzymes that promote inflammation in the body, which is associated with so many disease risks.

In addition to cutting down on processed foods, the collective wisdom on dieting also tells you to cut back on sugar, eat more vegetables and drink more water. This is all good, basic advice and you'll be following it on The Programme. But we're taking it to the next level, because I don't want you to eat just to lose weight, I want you to eat whole, real, powerhouse foods in combinations that fuel your inner athlete and help you become healthy and well. I've paired specific menu plans with specific types of workouts to help you optimise your performance, boost your metabolism and promote your health. The bottom line is that what you eat and how you move can keep your blood sugar levels under control, decrease inflammation in your body, and make you feel good. There are properties in specific foods, spices and herbs that can optimise your body for health, and The Programme is going to help you incorporate them into your diet too.

TAKING CHARGE

Worldwide, obesity has nearly doubled since 1980. In the UK, one in four adults is obese, and more than 60 per cent are either overweight or obese. Even young children are increasingly suffering from obesity: it affects 19 per cent of children aged ten to eleven and about 10 per cent of children aged four to five.

A number of lifestyle factors are responsible for this growing problem; not least is the way we eat, of course. The average diet has more saturated fat, salt, added sugar and refined grains than experts tell us are healthy – and less than the recommended amounts of vegetables, fruit, whole grains and dairy. Did you start your day with a standard breakfast cereal or toast and marmalade with juice and coffee, followed with a lunch of a sandwich made with white bread, ham and cheese, and crisps, and then have a couple of slices of pizza with a side salad for dinner? If so, you're not the only one. And you can do – and feel – so much better.

Most of us don't work up a sweat often enough either. Are you moving for at least 20 minutes every day? Many of us now spend more than seven hours a day sitting in front of TV, computer and mobile device screens and in cars, buses and trains.

You know why this is a problem. Being overweight puts you at an increased risk of heart disease, diabetes and certain kinds of cancer, among other things. It lowers your life expectancy and is likely to increase your insurance costs – and adds to the burden on our overstretched health service. And if you are carrying more weight than you need, you probably don't feel your best day-to-day. Now, it's possible to be overweight and relatively fit. Only you know where you are and where you want to be in terms of your weight. The Programme can help you lose weight, but I want to be clear: this isn't about you getting thin, it's about you getting strong, being healthy and feeling well in your body, for the rest of your life.

A better way to eat

Eating on The Programme means eating mindfully. It means paying attention to the ratio of lean protein, good carbohydrates and healthy fat in the foods you eat. I'm going to make it very easy for you to do that: you can use my recipes and meal plans or swap foods with things that work for you and your family. There is no category of food that is completely off limits, but I've provided lists of better choices within major food categories that you can use to help make your own decisions. As you assess the way you feel when you start eating to promote your health and performance, I'm betting it will get easier and easier to make the best choices.

Eating mindfully on The Programme also means paying attention to *when* you eat. Don't worry, I'm not going to tell you to eat at a particular time of day or that you can't eat certain food groups after breakfast or anything like that. The Programme is meant to fit into your life the way you want to live it. But this is also your new life, one that involves moving more, as a commitment to yourself and your well-being. To optimise your workouts, think about how and when you are going to exercise each day, because that is going to help you make your best eating choices.

WHAT YOU EAT

There are four types of Eat days on The Programme: Cleanse, Burn, Build and Relax – which are related to the type of physical activity you do on different days. (More about different types of exercise in the next chapter, Sweat.) During the next few weeks, you're going to follow them in the order that I've developed for The Programme, but once you complete this cycle and get the hang of eating this way you can choose your days as they work best for you. You will never need to leave The Programme to eat 'normally', or get bored following one routine endlessly – it's very flexible.

Cleanse The Programme starts with four Cleanse eating days to prime your body for what is to come. This is not a 'detox' or a 'cleanse' in the sense that you have probably heard those terms before. On a Cleanse day, you're going to eat light, eat clean and give your digestive system a bit of a break. This is not a fast and you will not be hungry. You'll be getting plenty of calories from nutrient-rich smoothies and soups, to help you work out. The recipes I'm recommending for these particular days include foods that have some evidence-based properties for healing the body and strengthening the immune system in various ways. I call these foods and their properties the 'Core Four' (see page 56) and you can incorporate them into your diet during other days as well.

Burn Unless you are already fairly active, you are probably going to move more on The Programme and you need to fuel yourself properly with the right ratio of complex carbohydrates to protein. You'll be eating slightly more carbohydrates on the days when you are burning energy in cardiovascular workouts.

You can tailor the meal plans depending on the time of day you train so that you can get the most out of your workouts. Particular combinations of certain types of protein, carbohydrates and fats are easier for your body to digest, so I have recommendations for how to adjust your plate depending on whether you're eating a particular meal before or after working out.

Build Building muscle and getting strong are critical parts of The Programme and, while you need protein every day (with every meal, actually), eating the right kind and amount of protein after strength training helps your muscles repair and develop in an optimal way. Build days have slightly more protein than days when you're doing Burn workouts. You'll eat to build, literally feeding your muscles, on the days that you focus on strength training, and you'll be paying attention to when and what you're eating relative to when you work out to maximise the relationship between your food and your workout.

Relax I struggled with what to call this day, because I hope you'll be calm and relaxed most of the time on The Programme, particularly in terms of your food. The body responds very quickly to being well nourished and I think you're going to like how you feel. But this is a day when you can relax your standards a little, and allow yourself something you wouldn't normally have on The Programme, such as a drink, a burger, a more calorie-dense dessert, or whatever part of your diet you enjoy, but has a limited place in a healthy diet. This is not a 'cheat' day, it's part of The Programme that recognises the realities of our lives, and helps you plan for them and incorporate them into an eating plan that does not derail your hard work. You should still work out on your Relax eating day, and how you choose to do that will determine how you plan to eat that day. I've provided an example of what a Relax day might look like for me so you can use it as a guide.

To kick-start The Programme you'll begin with four days of 'Cleanse' eating. For the next seventeen days you'll follow alternating 'Build' and 'Burn' meal plans. At the end of that, you'll experience a 'Relax' eating day. This chart sets it out as if you are starting on a Sunday, but you can begin The Programme on any day of the week.

Sun	Mon	Tue	Wed	Thur	Fri	Sat
Cleanse	Cleanse	Cleanse	Cleanse	Burn	Build	Burn
Build	Burn	Build	Burn	Build	Burn	Build
Burn	Build	Burn	Build	Burn	Build	Burn
Relax						

Once you've completed that cycle and are tuned in to this way of eating, you can repeat it or adjust it as it suits you. I have clients who schedule a Cleanse eating day once a week and other clients who only use a Cleanse day when they feel they need a bit of a reset. If you find that you are doing a lot of strength training, you may use the Build day eating plan more often. If you are primarily in a state of weight maintenance, you might allow yourself a Relax day more often than someone who is working hard to lose weight. The choice is yours, and the plan can be changed as your workouts change, as you grow stronger and as your goals evolve.

The differences between your Cleanse, Burn, Build and Relax days are subtle but real. They have to do with the ratio of protein to carbohydrates to fat in the meals you'll eat on those days, and when you eat them. Each type of eating day on The Programme is designed with a PCF ratio in mind (the percentage of food you eat during the day that is made up of protein, carbohydrates and fat) and you are going to start thinking about your overall diet in terms of these macro-nutrients.

Protein

Your body needs protein to supply the amino acids that it uses to build and repair muscle tissue and make essential enzymes and hormones. You also need it for energy and a well-functioning immune system. Depending on your size, you may be meeting your minimum requirements, but the benefits of higher protein intake are huge: it will help you build and maintain a leaner body that burns fat more efficiently and helps preserve muscle strength as you age. Most of you are going to be building muscle on The Programme and even if that isn't your main goal, I'm in favour of eating more protein and spacing it out over the day's meals and snacks. After you complete the four Cleanse days, you are going to eat protein at every meal.

The reason I advocate a higher protein intake is because research suggests that eating more protein when you are trying to lose weight helps you avoid losing lean muscle along with excess fat. Don't underestimate the satiety factor of protein-rich foods either: if you're getting used to eating less, protein will keep you feeling full, help reduce your appetite, and it actually requires your body to work a little harder to digest it compared to fat or carbohydrates, and this burns a few more calories. Many of my clients report being less likely to overeat protein compared to carbohydrate and fat.

It's generally best if most of your protein is lean. If you eat a lot of red meat or processed meats (sausages, salami, bacon and ham), that's got to change. Varying your diet to incorporate leaner and healthier sources of protein such as chicken and turkey, fish, eggs, pulses (beans, lentils, chickpeas), nuts and whole grains, will help you fuel up more efficiently and maximise the nutrients you're getting. Greek yogurt (which has a higher protein content than other yogurts), milk and cheese can also be good protein sources if you tolerate dairy foods. You can also use high-quality protein supplements in smoothies or to give other recipes a protein boost. Whey, egg, hemp and pea-based supplements are my preference. You will be expanding your repertoire of protein foods on The Programme; red meat does not have to be eliminated entirely (if you like it), but pay attention to the variety of different protein sources when you're planning your meals.

Carbohydrates

I know it's trendy to cut carbs if you're trying to lose weight, but not all carbs are the same, and the athlete in you can benefit from the good ones. Carbohydrates are the body's primary source of energy, and are needed for the healthy functioning of your kidneys, intestines, brain and central nervous system.

By now, you probably know what to do about carbohydrates if you're eating for health: you need to cut back on carbohydrates in the form of sugar and refined grains, like white bread, rice and pasta. That's not strictly about eating less, although you probably will if you cut right down on these foods, since they are so easy to overeat. It's really about their quality as energy sources: they're a quick source of energy but poor fuel. Eating refined carbohydrates causes a rapid rise in blood sugar, which triggers a large release of insulin in your body; insulin is a hormone responsible for storing excess sugar (glucose) from the blood; if your body doesn't need the glucose for energy, it gets stored in the form of extra fat.

But you don't need to cut all carbohydrates out of your diet in order to lose weight – and you shouldn't. Your muscles and your brain need glucose for energy, and you produce it when you digest carbohydrates. You just need to eat complex carbohydrates that your body will burn more slowly, and to eat them in combination with other foods that slow down their digestion. Complex carbohydrates – the kind found in fruits and vegetables, whole grains, pulses (beans, lentils, chickpeas), nuts, seeds, milk and yogurt – come with all kinds of vitamins, minerals and other vital nutrients. Most of them also contain fibre, which helps your digestive system function properly and makes you feel full, so you're likely to eat less. As a bonus, most non-starchy vegetables and fruits are relatively low in calories. If you commit to increasing the amount of fruit and veg in your diet as your primary source of carbohydrates, I can almost guarantee you'll be taking in fewer calories.

You can have complex carbohydrates at each meal or not, it's up to you, and your decisions can be made depending on when and how you're working out. When you choose healthy carbs – such as oats or quinoa – they will help keep your blood sugar stable, take longer to digest, and come with their nutrients intact. Just pay attention to the quantity you're eating and what you're eating them with.

Fat

You need to eat some fat. Period. It's another form of fuel for your body, and your most concentrated energy source. It maintains the health of your cell membranes, skin and hair, and is essential for some of your organs to function properly. Certain forms of fat can help reduce your risk for heart disease. Some key vitamins – A, D, E and K – are absorbed better with fat, so the nutritional benefit of a salad is improved by your using a little fat in the form of nuts, cheese or dressing. Fat tends to help you feel satisfied as well: it makes food taste good, which is important, and you digest fat a bit more slowly than carbohydrates, so it should keep you feeling full.

Fat is more calorie dense than protein and carbs (fat has 9 calories per gram; protein and carbs have 4) so you do have to watch your portions. The good news is that a little usually goes a long way.

There are different types of fat; the healthiest are unsaturated fats – from sources such as olive oil, high oleic sunflower and safflower oil, nuts, olives, avocados and oily fish such as salmon. Saturated fat, which tends to be solid at room temperature, is found in meat and poultry, butter, cream, cheese and chocolate; it can have a limited place in your diet on The Programme. Trans fats, which you are most likely to see in the form of partially hydrogenated oil, have been shown to increase your risk for heart disease and have no place in The Programme.

So, the combination of protein, carbohydrates and fat in your meals is what drives the food choices you'll make on The Programme, and the types of foods you use to supply those macronutrients will matter, but you have plenty of flexibility to plan meals that work for you and your family. Here are a couple of other things you'll need to pay attention to when you're making your food plans:

Sugar

Scientists tell us that refined sugar is an addictive substance: addictive in the same sense as alcohol or cigarettes, with associated health consequences. When you eat sugar – and refined carbohydrates are processed in your body in the same way as sugar even if they aren't sweet – your body experiences a sugar rush and then rapid depletion, like a drug high. What is happening is that your blood sugar spikes and then your body releases insulin to help your cells absorb that sugar. When that happens, your blood sugar drops back down and your body wants that rush all over again. The whole process happens quickly, like a roller coaster, especially if you haven't eaten protein and/or fibre with your sugar, which tend to slow the digestive process. The roller coaster of blood sugar highs and lows creates stress and inflammation in the body, and can leave you biochemically imbalanced. If you have ever seen your child come home on a high from a birthday party and then crash, you know what I'm talking about. As adults, we may become desensitised to those experiences in our own bodies but they are still happening, even if we have got used to them.

There is a system for ranking foods according to how quickly the body digests the carbohydrates in them: it's called the Glycemic Index (GI) and it can enhance your understanding of how your body experiences that sugar high. It's a useful tool, especially if you're concerned about your blood sugar (glucose) levels, and it can be really eye-opening to check the GI of certain refined or packaged foods that you enjoy. I don't like to get too hung up on this number, because most foods you'll be eating more of on The Programme have a naturally lower GI – and you can reduce the GI impact of a particular food by eating it in combination with protein, fat and/or fibre. The Programme generally follows the principal that eating lower on the GI scale is better, and that definitely means reducing sugar.

World Health Organization (WHO) guidelines recommend that adults and children limit their intake of so-called free sugars (not the kind that occurs naturally in whole fruit) to 6–10 teaspoons (25–40 grams) a day. If you track your sugar intake for a day or two before starting The Programme, you're probably going to find that you are exceeding that recommendation. Keep in mind that there are about thirty different ways sugar can be listed on an ingredients label!

When you do use added sugar, less processed forms of it, such as honey or real maple syrup, are better choices. I use raw manuka honey, which has active anti-inflammatory cultures, in my morning smoothies and sometimes in other recipes when I want them to be sweet. But it is still sugar, so it should be used sparingly. There is really no need for refined sugar (white or brown) on The Programme or in your diet. If that is going to be a radical change for you, try not to be overwhelmed but make small changes in the right direction before you start The Programme.

By the way, if a product that satisfies your sweet tooth is labelled low-sugar, reduced-sugar, no added sugar, light or calorie-free, it probably has artificial (chemically manufactured) sweeteners. These do not support your health. There are many types of artificial sweeteners and there is conflicting evidence about their safety and at what level they may inter-fere with healthy bacteria in your gut. I'm not a scientist. Here's what I know: these concentrated sweeteners, even if they turn out to be safe and help with weight loss or maintenance, are so intensely sweet that they distort your palate when you use them on a routine basis. When you eliminate them, or use them less often, you will honestly start to find naturally sweet things, like strawberries, more delicious and satisfying.

Stevia, because it is plant-based, would be my choice if you are going to use an artificial sweetener, and I've included it in a few of my recipes for people who want a bit of sweetness. But try to reduce your use of it gradually, and let your taste buds adjust. As a general rule, if you want to have something sweet to eat beyond a piece of fruit, I'd rather you ate a little bit of sweetness in a relatively natural state combined with a protein source. A plain yogurt mixed with a little fruit or honey is a better choice than a chemically flavoured, artificially sweetened, sugar-free, fat-free yogurt.

Fibre

Soluble fibre, which is found in some vegetables and fruit, pulses, oats and barley, has been shown to promote health and reduce the risk of heart disease and certain cancers. Insoluble fibre is a form of carbohydrate found in bran and wholemeal bread, the skins of vegetables and fruit, and in seeds and nuts. Although our bodies can't digest insoluble fibre, it helps your digestive system to function properly. Most people don't get enough of either type of fibre and overlook the role it can play in weight loss and in overall health.

Remember when I outlined the problem with foods that have a high GI? Fibre helps your body regulate the impact of such foods, by slowing down the rate at which sugar enters your bloodstream. It also aids your digestion by promoting healthy bacteria in your gut, prevents constipation, and can help reduce your cholesterol. Finally, because it's harder for your body to digest fibre, high-fibre foods keep you feeling full for longer, which will help you if you are adjusting to eating less.

Women should aim for 25 grams of fibre every day and men should ideally have 38 grams per day. I don't want to give you a lot of numbers to track but try looking at the fibre content of the foods you eat normally for a day or two. You'll probably be surprised at how little you get relative to the recommendations. See, I'm actually telling you to eat more of something!

Surprising serving sizes

In addition to paying attention to what kind of food you're using to fuel your body, you need to think about how much of it you eat. I don't know how tall you are, how old you are, how much you weigh, how much you want to weigh, or how active you are. These factors all affect how much you need to eat each day to function at your best.

Even if the food on your plate is very healthy, it is possible to have too much of it, and many of us have become confused about what 'full' should feel like. Everything seems bigger: our plates are oversized, we eat prepared foods more often (either as takeaways or in restaurants) and take advantage of 'supersized' food and beverage 'deals' when we shop. Most of us would benefit from learning about reasonable portion sizes and how to feel satisfied by them.

I think the easiest way to do this is downsize your dinner plate to something that's 19cm (7 inches) across – certainly no more than 23cm (9 inches) – and fill it according to the protein:carb:fat (PCF) ratio you are following for that meal. That might have half of it filled with non-starchy vegetables, a quarter of it filled with lean protein, and a quarter of it with a complex carbohydrate. Many people find using a smaller plate helps them control their portions without getting hung up on measurements or calories. If this might work for you, make sure you fill your plate in the kitchen and then bring that plate to the table, rather than serving the food in big 'help-yourself' dishes.

If you still feel hungry when your plate is empty, give yourself at least 20 minutes to evaluate your hunger before you decide to have seconds. Drink a glass of water, get up from the table, do something else in the meantime. Most people feel OK when they check back in after giving their brain a chance to 'catch up' with their stomach and register the feeling of being 'full'. If you decide that you are still hungry and are going to have more, you'll be making the choice in a conscious way.

To see if you are in tune with appropriate portion sizes, you can start educating yourself, as an exercise, by comparing the size of a serving on your favourite biscuits, cakes or sweets with how much you actually eat. That is usually eye-opening. A pack of biscuits generally gives nutrition information for a serving of one or two biscuits – but how often do you end up eating three or four?

Now, this works the other way too. For example, if I tell someone that they should really have eight servings of fruit and vegetables a day, they might say that they couldn't possibly eat that much. But if you understand that for most fruits and vegetables, a serving is about 85g (3oz), it seems much easier. The recommended serving sizes are a lot smaller than most people imagine, and they are often pleasantly surprised to realise how much fruit and veg they have been eating.

WHAT IS A SERVING?

Grains/Starches
1 slice of bread
30g (1oz) ready-to-eat cereal
60–70g (about 2½oz) cooked rice or pasta

Vegetables
2 good handfuls of raw leafy vegetables
85g (3oz) other vegetables
120ml (4fl oz) vegetable juice

Fruits
1 small fruit
140g (5oz) berries
120ml (4fl oz) fruit juice

Meat, poultry, fish, beans, nuts
55–85g (2–3oz) cooked lean meat, poultry or fish
150g (5oz) cooked dried beans or drained canned beans
2 tablespoons peanut butter

Milk, yogurt, cheese
240ml (about 9fl oz) low-fat milk or yogurt
40g (1½oz) low-fat cheese

Serving size cues

The recommended serving sizes are a lot smaller than most people think. If you don't want to bother measuring things out precisely every time, there are

➤

ways to visualize serving sizes: you'll get the hang of it quickly and it will soon become instinctive.

85g (3oz) meat = deck of cards or a computer mouse
85g (3oz) fish = cheque book
30g (1oz) cheese = four dice
1 cup = a small fist
8 tablespoons (½ cup) = tennis ball
4 tablespoons (¼ cup) = golf ball
1 tbsp = your thumb tip
1 tsp = your finger tip or one dice

You aren't going to be eating much packaged food on The Programme, but if and when you do, make sure you pay attention to the serving size on the food label. Things like nuts or granola, that might have a legitimate place in a healthy diet, can often be surprisingly calorie dense. I'm not asking you to count calories, but to tune in to what 'a serving' really is. Use measuring cups or spoons for a couple of days to get the hang of it – it may surprise you. The good news is that getting a more instinctive sense of how much you really need will help you choose food that is better fuel.

You have more control over your food when you prepare it at home. I like the convenience of eating out or ordering a takeaway just like you probably do, but restaurant portions tend to be much larger than any of us need and will usually have been prepared with larger quantities of oil or butter, for example, than you would use at home. Try to prepare your own food during the first cycle of The Programme, so that you know exactly what you're taking in. You'll also be adjusting your expectations: when you've been eating 'clean', your palate will become more sensitive to the heavier ingredients in meals, making it easier to resist larger quantities of them. And that will help you to make healthy choices.

One more thing

I know I'm talking about food as a form of fuel and in terms of macro- and micronutrients, but I want you to know that I understand that food is one of life's pleasures and it is one of mine. I love to eat. I care about food and how it tastes. I'm still evolving as a cook, but I enjoy creating breakfast smoothies and dinner scrambles, introducing my young son to new foods, and sharing great meals with my friends and family. My Sunday rituals include going to my local farmers' market. When I travel, I enjoy connecting with people who are growing and making food they care about. What we eat is both personal and social, and it needs to taste good in addition to being good for us. The Programme might change your diet but it doesn't have to change the fact that food can be a source of pleasure and meaning in your life. I hope you find that what you enjoy eating and how you enjoy it gets even better.

HOW YOU EAT

Begin with a Cleanse

Even though I'm calling these Cleanse days, please know that you are not dirty. The body has a very good system for cleaning and 'detoxifying' itself. But we give our bodies a hard task every day. Your liver, kidneys, colon and other systems are removing toxins from your organs, tissues and fat all the time. The way you're going to eat over the next few days will lighten their load a little bit and help prepare your body to make the most of all the nutrient-rich food you'll eat on The Programme. The digestive system is very important for your overall health and evidence suggests that gut health also plays a role in weight loss. The recipes for Cleanse days use ingredients that support your health in these key areas.

Everyone's experience is different, but some of my clients report that after eating in the Cleanse style for a few days they notice an improvement in their energy levels, concentration and skin condition, with less bloating, indigestion, sluggishness and headaches. Many of them experience weight loss. In other words, most of them feel better than they have been feeling. In addition to rebalancing your blood glucose and gut health, fighting inflammation in the body and burning some fat, eating 'clean' is also a good way to adjust your eating habits and practise a little discipline.

You are going to take a break from coffee, sugar, alcohol and dairy foods, and eliminate all processed food and animal protein over the next four days. Don't close the book! It's only four days. If you are very caffeine dependent, you might try eliminating or reducing your coffee or tea intake for a couple of days before starting The Programme, so that any effects of that withdrawal don't make the Cleanse days unpleasant for you. But some people choose to do it all cold turkey; it's up to you.

By the way, resist any temptation you might have to overeat the day before the Cleanse. Your aim is to reduce inflammation and bring your body back into balance and you're just going to make it harder on yourself if you go crazy the night before. This is not a fad diet and you're not permanently eliminating anything. And you may just have to trust me, but I think you're going to find that what you want to eat will change over time as you follow The Programme. But for now, if you're feeling anxious about it, just remind yourself that this is only four days and take it one day – or even one meal – at a time.

You are not going to be hungry because this is not a fast. The smoothies and soups will give you vitamins and minerals from fresh, raw, whole vegetables, fruits and nuts in a way that is easy for your body to digest and use. You will have plenty of calories and be able to exercise in the ways I suggest. Remember, this is not a crash diet, it's about feeling better. Moving will help you do that.

For the first four days, you are going to drink three smoothies and eat three soups each day. You can eat them in any order you want, just space them through the day. You can make all your smoothies and soups using the recipes I provide or you can substitute your own, as long as you follow my basic rules: the smoothies and soups must all contain three of the four essential elements – the 'Core Four' – that I describe below; and you need one vegetable-based soup and one bean-based soup each day. Otherwise, it's pretty flexible. You can choose which ones you want to make from the recipes I've provided for Cleanse days.

Smoothies

I love my morning smoothies and think they are an efficient, delicious way of starting the day. You're going to have three smoothies a day during the first four days of The Programme (the Cleanse days). You can make the same smoothie over and over again during those days or you can try all the recipes, it's up to you. I've offered 'upgraded' versions of the smoothies if you want to make them later in The Programme when you need more fuel (or if you're making them for people who aren't eating to Cleanse). If you want to buy or make a substitute smoothie, make sure it contains at least three of what I call the 'Core Four' elements. Also, although this is not really about counting calories, the Cleanse versions of the smoothies come in at around 200 calories per serving. If you're buying one, you need to keep that in mind. In most cases, I think you'll get more volume if you make one of my recipes. They're really easy!

Core Four for smoothies

Whichever smoothies you choose, you'll find yourself trying three of the Core Four:

Fit fats (unsaturated fats) Fat is your friend, at least the kinds I'm talking about. These include avocado, coconut, seeds, nuts, natural nut butters and the healthy fat (Omega-3) found in chia seeds and flax seeds (linseeds), as well as in fish such as salmon. Choosing these healthy fats, especially the Omega-3 sources, will help to reduce inflammation in the body, fuel your cells and keep your blood sugar in balance. These fats also help fight hunger, if you are eating less than you're used to during the Cleanse days.

Polyphenols Our bodies have molecules called free radicals that can cause a great deal of damage, especially to the arteries. Polyphenols are compounds, found in plants, that help prevent such damage. There is evidence that they act as antioxidants in the body and have potential health benefits, including reducing the risk of heart disease and cancer, and boosting good microorganisms in your digestive system. There are many different polyphenols, found in a variety of foods, including fruits and vegetables, spices and herbs (especially dried peppermint, cloves and star anise), cocoa powder (and dark chocolate), flax seeds (linseeds), coffee and green tea. Just-picked, fresh fruits and vegetables generally have higher levels of polyphenols than produce that's been sitting in your refrigerator for a while. Also, don't be too quick to peel: there is often a high concentration of polyphenols in the skin of fruit and veg.

Leafy greens These are loaded with antioxidants, vitamins and minerals. In addition to fighting inflammation, leafy greens are super-low in calories, and are a good source of fibre, which will help you feel fuller. Studies show that a little more than one serving of leafy greens daily can decrease your risk of diabetes by 14 per cent. If you don't already love the taste, many people find it easier to get their fill in a blended form; so if that's you, try the green smoothies. There are differences in the ways that greens taste, too. If you don't like iceberg or romaine lettuce, try rocket, watercress and butterhead. Try spinach, kale, Swiss chard, mustard greens, cavolo nero, cabbage and broccoli. Try them raw and cooked and in combinations with other ingredients until you find some favourites.

Power protein Protein powder and yogurt and/or kefir (a fermented milk drink, similar to yogurt) are the main protein sources for smoothies. Different types of protein powder are interchangeable in the recipes, but give whey-based proteins a try if you tolerate dairy (especially if you're drinking a smoothie later in The Programme, after a Build workout). Whey protein is generally easily digested and stimulates muscle growth. Seventy per cent of the immune system is in your gut. Yogurt and kefir contain probiotics that are important for gut health and help with immune function, so they are also good choices that you can use as your primary form of protein in the smoothies if you prefer. Emerging research also suggests an association between gut bacteria and weight, so the fermented dairy-based options offer this benefit as well. If you don't tolerate dairy (and even if you do,) pea- and hemp-based protein powders are good protein options; I suggest using a variety of vegetarian protein sources to ensure that you are obtaining all of the amino acids needed to make a 'complete' protein. There are many soy-based protein powders on the market; although you can use them in the smoothies, these aren't my preference because of emerging and conflicting evidence about other effects the overconsumption of soy can have in certain populations. Whey-, pea- and hemp-based powders don't seem to be raising the same concerns, so I'd encourage you to give them a try.

Soups

During the Cleanse days you eat three soups a day; at least one of them should be vegetable-based and one bean-based. You can make all of the soup recipes, and either use them during the Cleanse or freeze them to eat at any other point in The Programme. The recipes include suggestions for increasing their nutritional content or pairing them with other foods if you're cooking for family members who are not eating to cleanse.

If you want to create your own soups or buy ready-made options, that's fine, but each one must contain three of the 'Core Four' options for soup. Bean-based soups should contain approximately 200 calories per serving and vegetable soups should contain approximately 100 calories per serving. The recipes I provide (see Chapter 8) are very satisfying and fit that framework. Keep an eye on the serving size of anything you buy and if the equivalent seems small, try making one of mine.

Core Four for soups

Whichever soups you choose to make, they should include a combination of three of the following core elements, which I hope you'll keep incorporating into your diet throughout The Programme.

Spices and herbs Many contain polyphenols: bioactive compounds that some evidence suggests may help to reduce inflammation in the body. Sage, thyme, ginger, rosemary, marjoram and oregano have all been used for centuries as folk medicine, as have chilli pepper, black pepper and cinnamon. They taste great and add flavour and depth without adding fat or calories. The soup recipes in The Programme were developed to take advantage of these properties.

Cruciferous vegetables It is so worth developing a taste for these good guys – kale, cauliflower, cabbage, Brussels sprouts, pak choi, broccoli, rocket, swede, watercress. They are loaded with antioxidants, vitamins and minerals and are great fibre sources, which will help you feel fuller on Cleanse days. Some people find soups an easier way to incorporate these ingredients into their diet rather than eating them raw or steamed. You should try to eat some of these vegetables every day; most of the soups will cover this one for you.

Allium family Onions, garlic, shallots, spring onions, chives and leeks have been used for centuries for their health benefits. Research tells us that they contain organosulfides, a type of phytochemical, or plant compound, that is believed to have antioxidant properties. And of course these plants provide a rich flavour base for your soups (and many other meals) without added calories and fat. Onions have a higher polyphenol and flavonoid content than other members of the allium group, but you'll benefit from all of them.

Pulses (legumes) Kidney beans, black beans, white beans, chickpeas, lentils – you name it, they're all good! You can use my recipes or find recipes that have other types of pulses. Pulses are an excellent source of plant-based protein and fibre, which will help keep you full, and they contain antioxidants to help fight inflammation. There is also evidence that a daily serving of pulses may help reduce cholesterol and lower blood pressure. In addition, they are also generally a good source of magnesium, a mineral that most people don't get enough of. Pulses are also a slowly digested carbohydrate which helps keep blood sugar in check. The fact that they make satisfying and delicious meals is almost a bonus.

Sample Cleanse day

The smoothies and soups can be eaten in any order. I'd space them out and eat every two or three hours. Here are some suggestions for how your first Cleanse day might look:

Option 1	Option 2	Option 3
Java Mocha Smoothie	Green Tea Smoothie	Smoothie (Core 3)
Chocolate-covered Strawberry Smoothie	Cherry Almond Smoothie	Smoothie (Core 3)
Carrot and Ginger Soup	Tomato-Cucumber Gazpacho	Vegetable-based soup
Blueberry Pear Smoothie White Bean and Tuscan Kale Soup	Tropical Kale Smoothie Black Bean Soup with Pico de Gallo	Smoothie (Core 3) Bean-based soup
Carrot and Ginger Soup	Tomato-Cucumber Gazpacho	Vegetable-based soup

A couple of notes about Cleanse days

If you need to lose more than 23kg (50lb), are younger than 30, are a woman who is taller than 1.72m (5' 8"), or a man who is taller than 1.83m (6'), you can make one additional smoothie on Cleanse days and drink it at any point during the day.

If you are hungry between soups and smoothies, snack on Vegetable Stock (see page 253) or raw non-starchy vegetables – such as peppers, celery, cucumber, radishes, cauliflower, courgettes – in unlimited quantity. Some people find certain raw vegetables difficult to digest and part of the point of the Cleanse days is to let your digestive system take it easy, but if you're hungry and/or missing the 'crunch' from your food, feel free to snack on non-starchy vegetables that work for you.

All of the soup and smoothie recipes contain tips to increase calories and/or add protein so that you can use them later on in The Programme if you like them and want to make them even more substantial, depending on your workout.

BURN AND BUILD

After the first four days of The Programme, you'll start to ramp up your workouts: on some days the workout aims mainly to Burn fat, on others to Build strength. You'll need to adjust what you eat, according to the type of workout you're doing. You'll eat protein and fat at every meal; each day, you'll also eat at least:

Six servings of vegetables and fruit

One to two servings of dairy foods

Protein and fat at every meal

Burn day

On Burn days, you are going to eat with the aim of achieving a daily PCF ratio of 25/50/25. That means that your food over the course of the day should be made up of about 25 per cent protein, 50 per cent complex carbohydrates and 25 per cent fat. Don't worry, you don't need to calculate any of that. If you follow the meal plan, and as you'll see from the sample menu plan below and on page 64, I've done it all for you. Burn days include more grains and/or fruit. A sample Burn day might look like this.

Sample Burn day meal plan

BURN   PCF 25/50/25

Breakfast Breakfast Oat Cookies
1½ starches, 1 protein, 1 fruit, 2 fats

Lunch Chicken Caesar Wrap + carrots + 1 small orange
1½ starches, 3 protein, 1 fruit, 1½ vegetables, 1 fat

Snack 175g (6oz) fat-free plain Greek yogurt with 75g (2½oz) berries
1 dairy, 1 fruit

Dinner Sweet and Spicy Chicken Breast with Mashed Sweet Potato and Broccoli
1½ starches, 3 protein, 1½ vegetables, 1 fat

Optional Burn snack

Build day

On Build days, you'll be aiming for a PCF ratio of 30/40/30. That means that your food over the course of the day should be made up of about 30 per cent protein, 40 per cent complex carbohydrates, and 30 per cent fat. Again, don't worry, you don't need to calculate any of that. If you follow the plan, I've done it all for you, or given you the equivalent values so that you can substitute things without going off track. You'll notice one of your meals will not contain any grain or starch but that meal can have more protein and vegetables. Build days include particular protein-oriented snacks.

Sample Build day meal plan

BUILD   30/40/30

Breakfast Blueberry Chia Power Protein Pudding
1 dairy, 3 protein, ½ fruit, 2 fats

Lunch Salmon Salad Lettuce Wraps + grapes
1 starch, 3 protein, 1 fruit, 1½ vegetables, 1 fat, ⅓ dairy

Snack Cottage cheese and cherry tomatoes
1 dairy, 1 vegetable

Dinner Chicken Salad with Quinoa, Cucumber and Strawberries
1 starch, 4 protein, 1 fruit, 2½ vegetables, 1 fat

Optional Build snack

A couple of notes about Burn and Build days

While the PCF ratios for Burn and Build days are consistent, you'll notice, when you look at the meal plans (starting on page 68), that the food exchanges vary according to the sample menu. In other words, there are many different ways to get the correct balance of macronutrients in your day. The meal plans mix it up to keep it interesting, so make sure that if you substitute meals or snacks by using the exchanges, you actually use the ones for that particular meal or day.

Eating this way should not be a chore, and once you get used to it, it's pretty simple. You don't have to count calories or grams of anything. I have provided calorie counts in the sample meal plans, though, for those of you who do like to keep track of them, and so that you can understand how much you are eating. If you feel you need to eat more, depending on your meals and goals, you can adjust your portion sizes, either during your first cycle of The Programme or at any point in the future.

Notice that on both Burn and Build days, you'll be eating protein with every meal: 60–85g (2–3oz) at breakfast and 85–150g (3–5oz) at lunch and dinner. That's really important, both for feeling full and to protect and feed your muscle mass when you're working out. On Build days, you should have your protein-packed snack after your Build workout, preferably within 30 minutes.

If you need to lose more than 23kg (50lb), are younger than 30, are a woman who is taller than 1.72m (5' 8"), or a man who is taller than 1.83m (6'), you can eat an extra snack every day from the appropriate list and can feel free to add an additional ounce or two of protein per meal.

I've designed two 20-minute workouts for each day (more about this in the Sweat section beginning on page 82), but if you choose to do additional exercise on any day, so that your total amount of time spent working out is 90 minutes or more, you should also have an additional snack, regardless of your size.

RELAX DAY RULES

On the last day of the first cycle of The Programme, I introduce what I'm calling a Relax eating day. The reality is that food is not only fuel, it is a source of pleasure, and a way of celebrating and connecting with people you care about. Any realistic eating plan makes room for that in your life. The key is not to let that relaxing undo the benefits you gained from being disciplined about your eating and workouts or to derail your motivation to keep going. I see clients struggle with both of those challenges. Here's my best advice. Choose what kind of workout you want to do on your Relax day: it can be one of my Burn or Build workouts that you particularly enjoyed, or it can be something else that you love to do or want to try. You can go for a hike, a bike ride, a run, go kayaking, ice skating, play tennis or foot-ball, anything you might look forward to but do not have time to explore during a normal day. I know your life is busy, and the regular workouts on The Programme are designed to be about 20 minutes of maximum effort to fit into a crowded schedule. I'm imagining a Relax day to be one where you may have a bit more time and space to try other ways of moving that inspire you.

Choose your basic eating plan for your Relax day based on the type of workout you choose to do (is it more of a Burn or a Build?) and eat on-plan for the majority of the day but, if you want to, add a reasonable treat to your menu. For me, that might be a burger and a beer, both things I love but wouldn't eat on a daily basis. I don't know what you'll want: it could be a glass of wine, a dessert, a pasta dish, white bread. Whatever it is, be intentional about it. Make it something you really want and keep your portions reasonable. Be clear with yourself: the calories from alcohol or chocolate cake are not offering you nutritious fuel. They are satisfying another function, one that has a place in your life, but that stays in check if you want to be healthy.

Now, what if you go a little crazy and relax your eating plan beyond what you planned? This happens and it's a live-and-learn situation. Notice if there is a pattern to the types of foods or situations that challenge your discipline, and keep it in mind. The most important thing is to recommit to The Programme. For some of my clients, that might mean repeating a Cleanse day, in whole or in part. You do not have to do this, you can just rotate right back into a Burn or Build schedule of eating. But if you feel your motivation waning in the wake of a Relax meal or day, take action and head back to the Cleanse menus. For example, if you had a piece of cake on your Relax day, maybe you want to replace one meal tomorrow with one of the

Cleanse smoothies. If you had a glass of wine with that piece of cake, maybe you want to swap two meals from your next day with a Cleanse smoothie or soup. If you have three or more 'treats' during your Relax day, consider following up with a full Cleanse day from the beginning of The Programme.

What counts as a treat?

- Alcohol

- Extra starch serving (pasta, bread, chips, etc.)

- Refined grains

- Dessert or sweets

- Foods containing high amounts of fat (fried food, cheese plate, etc.)

PAYING ATTENTION

Most of us eat too quickly and don't pay much attention to our food. It takes about 20 minutes for the brain to register that our stomach is full, so when we eat quickly and mindlessly, it's easy to overeat before we get that message. We also tend not to fully appreciate or enjoy what we're eating when we're distracted. So, turn off your TV, put your phone in its charger, and try to really pay attention to your next meal.

Use my menu plans to reset your appetite, your palate and your body. I've given you the food exchanges and calorie counts for each meal to make it as easy as possible for you to switch ingredients or meals for things that are more appealing to you. These numbers are approximate and rounded, they are meant to give you general guidance and ease your ability to stay on track with The Programme when you want to eat differently.

But I hope you'll challenge yourself to try some new things during this time, and experiment with ways of incorporating healthy food into your diet. Don't give up on anything right away, especially if it's in one of the Core Four families. Try other strategies. For example, if you don't like kale raw in a salad, try blending it in a smoothie, or cooking it in a small amount of a healthy fat, with a spice that appeals to you. The menu plans that follow are just an example. Use them as building blocks to eat well forever – it all needs to taste good to you.

DAY BY DAY

The meal plans that follow show one way that The Programme can work, but remember that it's flexible: you can exchange ingredients (as explained on page 306) and you can swap the recipes with others from another day, as long as it is in the same category of day, i.e. another Build or Burn day.

DAY 1 CLEANSE   1019 calories

Java Mocha Smoothie	1 dairy, ½ fruit, 1 fat	192
Carrot and Ginger Soup	3 vegetables, ½ fat	128
Green Tea Smoothie	3 protein, 1 fruit, ½ vegetable, 1 fat	200
Blueberry Pear Smoothie	1 dairy, 1 fruit, ½ vegetable, 1 fat	211
White Bean and Tuscan Kale Soup	1 starch, 1 protein, 2+ vegetables, ½ fat	160
Carrot and Ginger Soup	3 vegetables, ½ fat	128
Fitness Assessment		
Slow-burn Cardio		

DAY 2 CLEANSE   1014 calories

Green Tea Smoothie	3 protein, 1 fruit, ½ vegetable, 1 fat	200
Cherry Almond Smoothie	3 protein, 1 fruit, ½ vegetable, 1 fat	220
Tomato and Cucumber Gazpacho	2 vegetables, 1 fat	92
Chocolate-covered Strawberry Smoothie	3 protein, 1 fruit, 1 fat	160
White Bean and Tuscan Kale Soup	1 starch, 1 protein, 2+ vegetables, ½ fat	206
Carrot and Ginger Soup	3 vegetables, ½ fat	128
Fitness Assessment		
Slow-burn Cardio		

DAY 3 CLEANSE   1030 calories

Blueberry Pear Smoothie	1 dairy, 1 fruit, ½ vegetable, 1 fat	211
Java Mocha Smoothie	1 dairy, ½ fruit, 1 fat	192
Curried Cauliflower Soup	2 vegetables, 1 fat	103
Tropical Kale Smoothie	1 dairy, 1 fruit, ½ vegetable, 1 fat	200
Black Bean Soup with Pico de Gallo	1½ starches, 2 protein, 2 vegetables, ½ fat	220
Mushroom and Pak Choi Soup	3 vegetables, ½ fat	104
Fitness Assessment		
Slow-burn Cardio		

DAY 4 CLEANSE   957 calories

Cherry Almond Smoothie	3 protein, 1 fruit, ½ vegetable, 1 fat	220
Chocolate-covered Strawberry Smoothie	3 protein, 1 fruit, 1 fat	214
Green Tea Smoothie	3 protein, 1 fruit, ½ vegetable, 1 fat	200
Black Bean Soup with Pico de Gallo	1½ starches, 2 protein, 2 vegetables, ½ fat	220
Curried Cauliflower Soup	2 vegetables, 1 fat	103
Fitness Assessment		
Slow-burn Cardio		

In the following meal plans B = Breakfast, L = Lunch, S = Snack and D = Dinner

DAY 5 BURN   1220 calories

Wake-up Workout B: Upgraded Green Tea Smoothie	3 protein, 2 fruits, 1 vegetable, 2 fats	290
L: Mexican Scramble	1½ starches, 1 vegetable, 2 fats, 4 protein, 1 fruit	410
S: 175g (6oz) fat-free plain or vanilla Greek yogurt with 75g (2½oz) berries	1 dairy, ½ fruit, 1 fat	180
D: Prawn Stir-Fry	2 starches, 3 protein, 2 vegetables, 2 fats	340
BURN Workout		

Exchanges for day: 3½ starches, 1 dairy, 10 protein, 3½ fruits, 3½ vegetables, 7 fats

DAY 6 BUILD   1270 calories

Wake-up Workout		
B: Power Protein Pancakes	1½ starches, ½ dairy, 2½ protein, ½ fruit	350
L: Quinoa Chicken Salad + 1 small peach	1½ starches, 4 protein, 1 fruit, 2 vegetables, 1 fat	410
S: 1 Babybel Light cheese and 15–16 whole almonds	1 dairy, 1 fat	160
D: Turkey Wraps and Salad	4 protein, 4 vegetables, 2 fats	360
BUILD Workout		

Exchanges for day: 3 starches, ½ dairy, 10½ protein, 1½ fruits, 6 vegetables, 4 fats

DAY 7 BURN   1330 calories

Wake-up Workout

B: Oatmeal Chia Porridge	1½ starches, 1 dairy, 3 protein, ½ fruit, 1 fat	410
L: California Turkey Wrap + 125g (4½oz) carrots + 175g (6oz) honeydew melon	1½ starches, 3 protein, 1 fruit, 2 vegetables, 1 fat, 1+ dairy	450
S: 2 small kiwi fruit and 7 walnut halves	1 fruit, 1 fat	180
D: Baked Pork Chop with Roasted Sweet Potato and Brussels Sprouts	1½ starches, 3 protein, 1½ vegetables, 1 fat	290

BURN Workout

Exchanges for day: 4½ starches, 2+ dairy, 9 protein, 2½ fruits, 3½ vegetables, 4 fats

DAY 8 BUILD   1250 calories

Wake-up Workout

B: Pumpkin Smoothie	1 dairy, 3 protein, 1 fruit, 1 fat	340
L: Tuna Spinach Salad + 1 small pear	1 starch, 4 protein, 1 fruit, 1½ vegetables, 1 fat	390
S: 75g (2½oz) steamed edamame beans	2 protein	120
D: Fajita Salad	1 starch, 4 protein, 3½ vegetables, 1 fat	400

BUILD Workout

Exchanges for day: 2 starches, 1 dairy, 13 protein, 2 fruits, 5 vegetables, 3 fats

DAY 9 **BURN** 1220 calories

Wake-up Workout

B: Breakfast Oat Cookies	1½ starches, 1 protein, 1 fruit, 2 fats	310
L: Chicken Caesar Wrap + 60g (2oz) carrot sticks + 1 small orange	1½ starches, 3 protein, 1 fruit, 1½ vegetables, 1 fat	420
S: 175g (6oz) fat-free plain Greek yogurt with 75g (2½oz) berries and stevia (optional)	1 dairy, 1 fruit	140
D: Sweet and Spicy Chicken Breast with Mashed Sweet Potato and Broccoli	1½ starches, 3 protein, 1½ vegetables, 1 fat	350

BURN Workout

Exchanges for day: 4½ starches, 1 dairy, 7 protein, 3 fruits, 3 vegetables, 4 fats

DAY 10 **BUILD** 1285 calories

Wake-up Workout

B: Upgraded Java Mocha Smoothie	1+ dairy, 2 fruits, 2 fats	310
L: Turkey Mushroom Scramble + ½ savoury muffin	1 starch, 4 protein, 1½ vegetables, 2 fats	330
S: 60g (2oz) lean cold meat + 1 apple	2 protein, 1 fruit	255
D: Salmon, Roasted Beetroot and Goat Cheese Salad + wholemeal roll	1 starch, ½ dairy, 4 protein, 2 vegetables, 1 fat	390

BUILD Workout

Exchanges for day: 2 starches, 1½+ dairy, 10 protein, 3 fruits, 3½ vegetables, 5 fats

DAY 11 BURN

1210 calories

Wake-up Workout

B: Upgraded Blueberry Pear Smoothie	1 dairy, 1½ protein, 2 fruits, 1 vegetable, 1 fat	320
L: Chicken Caprese Wrap + 150g (5oz) grapes	1½ starches, 2 protein, 1 dairy, 1 fruit, 2 vegetables	390
S: 1 small banana + 1 tbsp natural peanut butter	1 fruit, 1 fat	200
D: Sautéed Prawns with Broccoli + Rice	1½ starches, 4 protein, 1½ vegetables, 1 fat, ½ dairy	300

BURN Workout

Exchanges for day: 3 starches, 2½ dairy, 7½ protein, 4 fruits, 4½ vegetables, 3 fats

DAY 12 BUILD

1225 calories

Wake-up Workout

B: Baked Egg 'Muffins' + 1 small orange	½ dairy, 2½ protein, 1 fruit, ½ vegetable	260
L: Buffalo Chicken Salad + 150g (5oz) strawberries	1½ starch, ½ dairy, 4 protein, 1 fruit, 1½ vegetables, 1 fat	420
S: 175g (6oz) fat-free plain or vanilla Greek yogurt with 2 tbsp sunflower seeds	1 dairy, 1 protein, 2 fats	190
D: Turkey Meatballs and Tomato Sauce with Courgette Noodles	1 starch, 4 protein, 4 vegetables, 1 fat	355

BUILD Workout

Exchanges for day: 2½ starches, 2 dairy, 10½ protein, 2 fruits, 6 vegetables, 4 fats

DAY 13 BURN   1325 calories

B: Peanut Butter and Egg White Porridge with Blueberries	2 starches, 1½ protein, 1 fruit, 2 fats	350
L: Turkey Wrap with Veggies + 1 small apple	1½ starches, 1+ dairy, 2 protein, 1 fruit, 3 vegetables	420
S: 1 small orange and 1 hard-boiled egg	1 protein, 1 fruit	130
D: 90g (3oz) Steak with Beetroot and Green Beans	3 protein, 1½ vegetables, 2 fat	425
BURN Workout		

Exchanges for day: 3½ starches, 1+ dairy, 4½ protein, 3 fruits, 6 vegetables, 4 fats

DAY 14 BUILD   1310 calories

Wake Up Workout		
B: Baked Avocado with Egg White	2 protein, 1 fruit, 2+ fats	290
L: Chicken Bean Lettuce Wraps + veggies + 175g (6oz) cantaloupe melon	1 starch, 4 protein, 1 fruit, 3 vegetables, 1 fat	420
S: 60g (2oz) lean prosciutto	2 protein	160
D: Salmon Cakes with Dill Sauce and Roasted Asparagus	1 starch, 1 dairy, 4 protein, 3 vegetables, 1 fat	440
BUILD Workout		

Exchanges for day: 2 starches, 1 dairy, 12 protein, 2 fruits, 6 vegetables, 4+ fats

DAY 15 BURN   1320 calories

Wake Up Workout

B: 1 slice wholemeal toast topped with 1 tbsp natural peanut butter + 75g (2½oz) blueberries + 1 whole egg + 1 egg white, hard-boiled	1 starch, 1 fruit, 2 protein, 1 fat	390
L: Chicken, Bean, Rice and Avocado Bowl + 2 kiwi fruit	2 starches, 4 protein, 1 fruit, 1 vegetable, 1 fat	430
S: 175g (6oz) fat-free plain or vanilla Greek yogurt with 75g (2½oz) berries	1 dairy, 1 fruit	130
D: 90g (3oz) Salmon with 60g (2oz) Quinoa and 150g (5oz) Asparagus	1 starch, 3½ protein, 3 vegetables, 1 fat	370

BURN Workout

Exchanges for day: 4 starches, 1 dairy, 9½ protein, 3 fruits, 5 vegetables, 3 fats

DAY 16 **BUILD**   1270 calories

Wake-up Workout

B: Blueberry Chia Power Protein Pudding	1 dairy, 3 protein, ½ fruit, 2 fats	370
L: Salmon Salad Lettuce Wraps + handful of grapes + 60g (2oz) carrots	1 starch, 3 protein, 1 fruit, 1½ vegetables, 1 fat, ⅓ dairy	350
S: 115g (4oz) low-fat cottage cheese and 150g (5oz) cherry tomatoes	1 dairy, 1 vegetable	140
D: Chicken Salad with Quinoa, Cucumber and Strawberries	1 starch, 4 protein, 1 fruit, 2½ vegetables, 1 fat	410

BUILD Workout

Exchanges for day: 2½ starches, 1⅓ dairy, 10 protein, 2½ fruits, 5 vegetables, 4 fats

DAY 17 **BURN**   1365 calories

Wake-up Workout

B: Breakfast Tortilla + 175g (6oz) strawberries	1½ starches, ½ dairy, 2 protein, 1 vegetable, 1 fruit, 1 fat	395
L: Tortilla Pizza with Green Salad	1½ starches, 2 protein, 3 vegetables, 1 fat	360
S: Small pear and 2 Laughing Cow Light triangles	1 dairy, 1 fruit	160
D: Chicken and Vegetable Kebabs with Tzatziki + rice	1 starch, 1 dairy, 3 protein, 2 vegetables, 2 fats	450

BURN Workout

Exchanges for day: 4 starches, 2½ dairy, 7 protein, 1 fruit, 6 vegetables, 4 fats

DAY 18 BUILD   1205 calories

Wake-up Workout

B: 1 slice wholemeal toast, 175g (6oz) cottage cheese, 175g (6oz) chopped tomato, ½ grapefruit + 1 tsp butter (for toast, if desired)	1 starch, 3 protein, 1 fruit, 1 vegetable, 1 fat	330
L: Greek Chicken Salad	3 protein, 1 dairy, 2 vegetables, 1 fat	330
S: 175g (6oz) fat-free plain or vanilla Greek yogurt with 1 tbsp sunflower seeds	1 dairy, 1 fat	140
D: 115g (4oz) grilled steak with 100g (3½oz) steamed green beans (in 1 tsp olive oil), ½ baked sweet potato + 1 tsp butter (if desired)	1 starch, 4 protein, 3 vegetables, 2 fats	405

BUILD Workout

Exchanges for day: 2 starches, 2 dairy, 10 protein, 2 fruits, 6 vegetables, 5 fats

DAY 19 **BURN** 1200 calories

Wake-up Workout

B: Upgraded Tropical Kale Smoothie	1+ dairy, 2 fruits, 1½ vegetables, 1 fat	290
L: Greek Chicken and Veggie Pitta + cucumber + 2 clementines	1 starch, 3 protein, 1 fruit, 1½ vegetables, 1 fat	340
S: 1 small banana + 1 tbsp natural peanut butter	1 fruit, 1 fat	180
D: Chicken Veggie Pasta	1½ starches, 3 protein, 1½ vegetables, 1 fat	390

BURN Workout

Exchanges for day: 2½ starches, 1+ dairy, 6 protein, 4 fruits, 4½ vegetables, 4 fats

DAY 20 **BUILD** 1290 calories

Wake-up Workout

B: Ham and Veggie Scramble and Toast + 175g (6oz) honeydew melon	1 starch, 3 protein, ½ dairy, 1 fruit, 2 vegetables, ½ fat	370
L: Chicken Tacos	4 protein, ½ vegetable, 2 fats	310
S: 175g (6oz) fat-free plain or vanilla Greek yogurt and 1 tbsp sunflower seeds	1 dairy, 2 fats	200
D: Portobello Beef Burger and Courgette Fries with Tomato Sauce	1 starch, 4½ protein, 4 vegetables, 1 fat	410

BUILD Workout

Exchanges for day: 2 starches, 1½ dairy, 11½ protein, 1 fruit, 5½ vegetables, 5½ fats

DAY 21 BURN   1290 calories

Wake-up Workout

B: Nut and Berry Cereal Parfait + hard-boiled egg	1 starch, 1+ dairy, 1½ protein, ½ fruit, 1 fat	370
L: Turkey Burger and Green Salad + 2 kiwi fruit	2 starches, 3 protein, 1 fruit, 2 vegetables, 2 fats	460
S: 150g (5oz) grapes and 1 Babybel Light cheese	1 dairy, 1 fruit	130
D: Chicken Fajitas	1½ starches, 3 protein, 2½ vegetables, 1 fat	330

BURN Workout

Exchanges for day: 4 starches, 2+ dairy, 7½ protein, 2½ fruits, 4½ vegetables, 4 fats

DAY 22 RELAX

We all have foods or drinks we enjoy but that we know need to have a limited role in a healthy diet. Any plan has to make room for them if you're going to stick to it over the long haul. Now, we all crave different things, so I'm not sure what your relax day might look like. But I can show you one of mine, so that you can get a sense of what relax means … enjoy, but don't go crazy! It's really easy to undo a week's worth of self-discipline about eating and exercise. That's why I wait so long in The Programme before suggesting a relax day: I'm hoping, at this point, that you'll be satisfied with relatively modest indulgence. This is an optional day at this point in The Programme. I don't know what's going on in your life or what your goals are, but you can use the previous 21 days as a guide to help you keep moving towards them. But I know there are going to be days when you want to celebrate, take it easy and enjoy. This is what that might look like.

DAY 22 Jessie's RELAX DAY

Wake-up Workout

B: Green drink + Greek yogurt + berries	Cucumber, kale, avocado, lemon, lime, cayenne, cider vinegar
L: Green eggs scramble	Eggs, turkey, green pepper, avocado, tomato, cayenne
S: Chicken with spicy avocado	Grilled chicken, avocado, bean sprouts, vegan mayo, cayenne, Greek pepperoncini (hot peppers, from a jar)
D: Burger, beer, salad	

Weekend Challenge Workout
and/or a hike

CHAPTER 4

SWEAT

··

The quality of your food, and how much of it you eat, is a critical component of your health. But you can be at a healthy weight and follow a 'perfect' diet and still not be physically fit. As human beings, we were all designed to move, and if there is a better way to improve your overall quality of life than moving more, I don't know what it is. Many of us live from the neck up, but exercise allows us to live through our whole bodies. When I don't work out regularly, I honestly miss it. If that is not a feeling you can identify with, I wonder if you have fully committed to exercise in the past. You may not like the gym – and that's fine – but once you stick with a workout routine and find a type of exercise that you enjoy, it really changes you. Everyone I have ever worked with who has done this has got the bug. You have to commit to your workout and keep trying exercise options to find what you like, but it's well worth it. By the time you've done The Programme, a daily sweat will be as routine for you as eating and sleeping. Believe it or not, you're going to look forward to it and feel great.

THE WHY OF EXERCISE

Even if you haven't yet experienced how good exercise can feel, you know it's good for you. Being disciplined means doing things we know are important or good for us even when we don't want to do them. But if you're still at the stage where you find working out awkward or challenging, it will help you stay disciplined if you know *why* exercise is so good for you and can connect that knowledge to your personal motivation. So, if working out isn't already fun for you (and it will be, if you give it a little time), know that regular physical activity will directly improve your well-being in surprising ways.

- **Exercise improves your physical health**
  Different types of regular exercise can make you stronger and faster, improve your flexibility and agility, and make your body more efficient and functional. People who exercise regularly have better heart health, blood pressure, cholesterol levels, fewer neurological and memory-related problems, are less likely to have cancer, and generally live longer compared with people who don't move a lot. A sedentary lifestyle is associated with a greatly increased risk of death from cardiovascular disease and a number of other illnesses. You don't have to sweat hard to benefit from exercise: just 30 minutes of moderate activity (like brisk walking) each day is associated with a reduced risk of diabetes, heart disease and certain types of cancer. But there are benefits to pushing further for strength: most adults begin to lose muscle mass at up to one per cent a year after the age of twenty five. Weight training can curtail that loss, strengthen your bones and keep you stronger, and less injury-prone, for longer. Everyone can benefit from moving more and challenging themselves, but if you have been completely

inactive, there is great news: you have the most to gain from starting a regular exercise programme. It's not too late!

● **Exercise helps you get to and maintain a healthy weight**
Regular exercise does not give you carte blanche to have a poor diet. What and how much you eat has a huge influence on how much you weigh. But burning calories during exercise does allow you to eat a little more without gaining weight, and will certainly help you lose weight when you control your diet and exercise regularly.

There is nothing like the feeling of a good sweat after a long, hard workout and one of the great benefits, especially if you push at the end of a session, is something called an 'after burn', which means your metabolism is working harder for a time post-exercise. If your exercise periods are broken up into smaller sessions throughout the day, you'll be boosting your metabolism more often and getting that after burn multiple times, so that is one advantage to incorporating activity throughout your day. The Programme workouts are designed with this in mind.

People who want to lose weight often focus on the cardio forms of working out, but strength training to help build and keep lean muscle mass is critical: muscle burns more calories than body fat, which raises your metabolism and helps you burn more when you're not exercising.

Regular exercise is also hugely important in preventing weight gain and maintaining weight loss. The clients I've worked with who have lost extreme amounts of weight do best back in the 'real world' when they stay active.

● **Exercise feeds your mind**
Regular aerobic exercise increases the flow of blood and oxygen to your brain, and stimulates chemicals in your brain that positively affect the health of your brain cells. The

evidence here is specifically for aerobic exercise, and it suggests that regular moderate activity can protect your cognitive functioning, regenerate nerve functioning in your brain and improve your verbal memory and your ability to process information. So it seems that exercise makes you smarter.

- **Exercise reduces feelings of stress**
  There is evidence that exercise can be as effective as therapy and meditation in helping people cope with stress. While it's natural for all of us to have periods of stress, many of us don't take it as seriously as a physical health issue. Stress can increase bodily inflammation, lower immunity, raise blood pressure, and generally make you feel anxious and unwell. I don't know of a better, cheaper, natural stress reliever than the endorphins (chemicals released by the brain) produced by exercise. Exercise won't just improve your mood, it will provide physiological benefits that improve your overall management of stress. It should also help you rest and sleep, which always makes things more manageable. When you are exhausted and out of breath at the end of a workout where you have given it your all, you are going to feel amazing. That's a serious reward to me, as much as any weight loss or improved body fat percentage.

- **Exercise helps you connect**
  Exercise doesn't just help you live longer, it helps you live *better*. Studies tell us that being active when you are older generally means you can be more independent, and people of all ages who are active usually have a greater sense of well-being than sedentary people. Physical activity is also a great way to meet other people. If you can find other people who like the same activities as you, it is likely to be a source of friendship and support, not to mention a great motivator for you to keep moving. When you exercise out of doors, it will

also help you connect to nature, which will support your mental well-being – I know it helps mine!

- **You are going to have so much fun**
  You don't have to be 'good' at an exercise to enjoy it. You do have to be game to get outside of your comfort zone and try different activities so that you can discover what you like. But I've yet to have a client who didn't eventually find something they felt good about doing. That's important because if it's not fun, you won't stick with an exercise programme, no two ways about it.

  Look, it's painful to push yourself and I don't know anyone who truly enjoys every minute of every workout, even though most people feel great afterwards. But you do need to find ways to move that you enjoy. Be patient. Don't be afraid to try lots of different things, and try not to be self-conscious about your skill level. Most people do well with a varied mix of workouts so that they don't get bored. It may take you a while to find what you truly love. I've had clients who preferred walking or hiking to running, and then evolved into runners after several years. I've also had clients who were committed cyclists, who started swimming in the winter when it was too cold to bike, and that became their primary form of cardio exercise even in peak cycling season. Someone I've worked with put on a pair of ice skates with her son last winter for the first time in fifteen years and is still skating once a week on her own. You just never know what is going to energise you. Sometimes what your body is looking for at a given moment will surprise you. Be open to it. Anything that keeps you active is positive.

HAVE I SOLD IT? LET'S GET STARTED

There is no magical secret. When you train properly, your body gets stronger, faster and better. There are also no shortcuts. If you train correctly, you'll see improvements quickly, but if you hit it too hard and exercise to the point of exhaustion, you'll get burned out, or, worse, injured. Your workouts should challenge you but at an appropriate pace for the long haul. That is different for everyone, and you'll spend some time during the first four days of The Programme assessing your fitness level so you can find the right workout for you.

Your training plan also needs balance and variety. The benefits of working out come from different forms of exercise. Everyone should want to strengthen their muscles, avoid disease and injury, and improve their cardiovascular health. Many of you also want to lose fat. These are related, but different, goals, and are best achieved by a mix of movements. Whatever your fitness level, on The Programme you'll be engaging in four different types of exercises to help you reach your goals efficiently.

During most of The Programme, the focus of your workouts alternates between 'Burn' days and 'Build' days. But the plan is designed to improve five key components of your physical fitness. During the next 21 days you will be training in a strategic way in order to increase your

- strength

- metabolic conditioning

- athleticism

- cardio endurance

- flexibility

You will be focusing on one of these elements at each workout.

Strength training (Build)

Strength training helps maintain muscle mass and protects bone health, reducing the risk of osteoporosis. As we age we lose muscle mass: some estimates indicate we lose between 2.5 and 3kg (5–7lb) of muscle each decade after the age of twenty. Strength training improves your ability to do everyday activities, like picking up your child or a bag of heavy groceries; these daily activities require strong muscles. More strength means you put less strain on your joints and reduce the risk of injuries.

Metabolic training (Burn)

Metabolic training is a form of high-intensity training. It uses compound exercises with just a little rest in between exercises and increases your metabolic rate during and after the workout. High intensity workouts require more energy from anaerobic (that means without oxygen) pathways; the 'afterburn' effect you get after working out like this is called EPOC (Excess Post-exercise Oxygen Consumption.) Basically, you continue burning calories even when you are not working out! High intensity interval training is efficient and effective, and you'll include a bit of it every day in your Wake Up workouts, but it's also challenging, so make sure you work at your own pace, especially if you are just getting started.

Athletic training (Burn)

Athletic training improves our agility, balance, speed and coordination. Agility is the ability to change direction quickly. Balance is our ability to maintain our equilibrium, whether we're moving or standing still. Speed means movements such as sprinting and rapid jumps. Coordination is the ability to control the movement of your body in cooperation with your sensory functions, for example catching a ball. I've designed particular workouts to focus on specific skills in each of these categories.

Cardio endurance training (Slow Burn)

Cardio endurance training involves continuous aerobic activity such as walking, jogging, biking, using an elliptical machine, or swimming. Unlike the metabolic and athletic training workouts that vary between high intensity and recovery intervals, it is carried out at a fixed intensity level and therefore is often called steady-state cardio. It will increase your endurance and improve your mood. Anytime you're in a bad mood, get out and walk or do one of these activities if you possibly can, you're likely to feel a lot better. This type of aerobic exercise also reduces the risk of many health problems, including obesity, heart disease, high blood pressure, type 2 diabetes and stroke.

Flexibility training (Flow)

Flexibility is the ability of our joints and muscles to move through their full range. Our level of flexibility is primarily due to our genetics, but we all lose flexibility as we age and need to maintain it with regular training. Being flexible improves our posture, reduces the risk of injury, improves athletic per-formance, and can help reduce stress. The yoga flow that you will be doing is designed to not only increase your flexibility and range of motion, but also to reduce stress and tension by helping you to focus consciously on your breath. You can use this short series of exercises as a cool-down after any of your Burn or Build workouts, or at any point that you want to work on increasing your flexibility and range of motion.

The Programme workouts have been designed to increase your fitness in all five of these areas and are balanced so that even though I'm asking you to work out every day, you shouldn't be straining or overusing any particular muscle area. The other cool thing about paying attention to these different ways of working out is that you should get a more nuanced understanding of areas of your own fitness and how they vary. Most of us are stronger in one area or another, and most of you will find something to feel really good about and something that challenges you. You will also become more knowledgeable about which types of training support your specific goals.

BEFORE YOU BEGIN

Get a check-up

Before you begin any new exercise regime, including The Programme workouts, it is important that you check with your doctor, especially if you haven't been active recently. Not all exercises are appropriate for everyone; you may need to modify some of the moves in The Programme based on your personal health issues.

Monitor your intensity

One of the most common mistakes people make is not measuring their exercise intensity. You need to have a sense of how hard you are working in different types of workouts. Working too hard can lead to injury and burnout, while not working hard enough can lead to frustration from lack of results. So keep track of your exercise intensity at every workout.

The most common ways to monitor exercise intensity is by target heart rate:

Heart rate

To monitor your heart rate you can either wear a heart rate monitor or measure your pulse periodically as you exercise. According to the American Medical Association, your maximum heart rate (MHR) is approximately 220 minus your age. Aim to stay within 50 to 85 per cent of your maximum heart rate; this range is called your target heart rate. There are various free target heart rate calculators online, or you can use the table below to calculate your target heart rate zone, or training zone. If you choose to do any of your slow-burn cardio walks or runs on a treadmill, it is likely to have a heart monitor function.

Moderate exercise intensity:
50 to 70 per cent of your maximum heart rate

Vigorous exercise intensity:
70 to 85 per cent of your maximum heart rate

If you're just starting out, aim for the lower end of your target zone (50 per cent). Then gradually increase your target zone.

Maximum heart rate and training zone, by age

Age	Maximum Heart Rate per Minute	Training Zone: 60% Rate	Training Zone: 80% Rate
20	200	120	160
25	195	117	156
30	190	114	152
35	185	111	148
40	180	108	144

Age	Maximum Heart Rate per Minute	Training Zone: 60% Rate	Training Zone: 80% Rate
45	175	105	140
50	170	102	136
55	165	99	132
60	160	96	128
65	155	93	124

Source: American Medical Association

Note Some types of medications can lower your maximum heart rate (and, therefore, lower your target heart rate zone). This is another good reason to check with your doctor – so you can ask them if you need to use a lower target heart rate zone because of any medications you take or medical conditions you have.

YOUR TRAINING SCHEDULE

The Programme is designed to improve your fitness in the five key areas described on page 87. In order to get fitter, however, you need to assess your current level of fitness.

Start with fitness assessments

In addition to training in various ways, you need to train at an appropriate level. You don't want to hurt yourself. But once you get started, you do want to feel challenged. Your muscles and performance respond to appropriate training stress, which means you need to up the ante from one series of workouts to the next in order to see improvement, otherwise your fitness will plateau. The beautiful thing is that your body is able to evolve and adapt to what you ask it to do. So be patient with your progress, but know that you need to push yourself. Listening to your body and finding that balance is key.

The first step on your 21-day transformation is to establish your fitness level in four key areas by taking some brief assessment tests. If the thought of that gives you a not-so-pleasant flashback to your school gym class, don't worry. These assessments are designed to give you an idea of what workouts are most appropriate to begin with and help you track your progress – you are in a judgement-free zone!

For the first four days of The Programme, while you are Cleanse eating, you're going to perform a few brief exercises each morning to evaluate your fitness level in one key fitness area and follow up with a gentle slow cardio workout (walking, running or some combination of the two) that is just meant to get you up and moving. The evaluations themselves are brief, so you can do the workout immediately after the fitness assessment, but you don't have to. It's fine to assess in the morning and work out at night if that fits your schedule. However, I like it when people start their day with exercise, because you can carry through the day that feeling of having given yourself the gift of health.

Each fitness assessment features a series of four exercises of the type I might get a new client to do in my gym to see where they're at. The main function of the assessments is to help you figure out whether you should start training at the Beginner, Intermediate or Advanced level (although, if you enjoy doing them, you may want to add them to your weekly routine). You can use these exercises to track your progress once in a while, too. You should repeat the assessments at the end of your first cycle on The Programme, and every month or so afterwards, so that you can adjust your fitness goals as you need to and also celebrate your progress. Don't worry if it turns out that you fall into different categories in different areas. You might be ready to do the Advanced strength workout but are more limited in your flexibility, so you will be doing the Beginner series on another day. That's fine.

Finding the right challenge

It's important to do some type of movement every day. Some of the workouts you'll be doing on The Programme are Tabata-influenced exercises (named after Dr Izumi Tabata, who discovered the effectiveness of this type of exercise), which are a form of high intensity interval training (HIIT). These are brief and intense bursts of exercise that burn calories and boost your metabolism, interspersed with periods of rest. You'll also need to try other new forms of exercise and strategies that will get you excited to move.

You are reading this book, so I know you're motivated. You may have some very big goals, that's good, but it can get overwhelming. Getting from here to there requires you to pay attention to one small decision at a time. If you're feeling panicky about how far you have to go, just commit to one workout at a time. Worry about your next workout after you finish this one. Don't go too hard and burn out or get injured.

Some clients get excited about starting a new exercise pro-gramme and think they need to do cardio exercise really hard and chase that 'burn' feeling. The enthusiasm is great, but if your muscles are not strong, you're going to wind up sweaty, sore, worn out and possibly too injured to do your next workout. That's no good. You need a training plan that improves your core stability, strength and agility, as well as your heart health, so you can get sweaty, sore and tired in the right way, to see maximum results. That means you need to mix up your work-outs, take the time to understand your body's reaction to them and, if necessary, slow down. Take things gradually.

Finding partners

You do not need to work out with other people. But there are tremendous benefits to exercising with a partner or a group, and I encourage you to seek out opportunities to do that during The Programme. Consider starting The Programme with a friend so that you can support each other. Explore the possibility of trying a fitness class or group workout. Working out with other people can give you the motivation to show up, plus you will receive healthy competition to perform at your best, friendship and encouragement from people who share your fitness goals and, sometimes, inspiration from people who are a little ahead of you. Having an exercise partner keeps you accountable and can also make the time pass more enjoyably. Finally, taking a class or working with a professional trainer can be stimulating – it's an easy way to mix up your fitness routine and can open your eyes to new ways of doing things.

If you have been put off gyms in the past or are new to them, don't be afraid to try out different ones. Gyms are like bars or other places that people gather. Most of them are very welcoming and thrilled to have people of all fitness levels, but one might feel more comfortable to you than another, so explore your options. Sometimes going with a friend can make it less intimidating, too, so see if you can round up an interested partner.

I love the people at my gym; they make it feel like home to me. But gyms are not your only possible fitness community. Think about what you liked to do when you were a kid. Did you play rugby or football? Find an adult league. Did you like riding your bike? There might be a group of weekend riders in your area. Did you dance? Sign up for a class; you'll probably still like it. Was there something you always wanted to try? This is your moment to make it happen. As you try out new ways of moving on The Programme, make some of it social if you can: you'll be much more likely to stick with it and you'll have more fun.

Stay in motion

Walk It might sound counterintuitive, but walking is a terrific choice if you're feeling tired and sore. Gentle movement of this kind will actually help you recover from general soreness more quickly than complete rest. It can also be energising. If you're feeling restless and want to keep moving, walking is great. Walking is not going to directly improve your performance at other activities and is not a tough enough exercise to build strength, but it is a low-to-no-impact way to burn calories, keep your blood flowing and your muscles moving, all without impacting your ability to hit it hard during your next workout. Walking also provides a restful mental reset. Little walks, long walks, doesn't matter: it all adds up and there's no downside to it. If in doubt, try walking it out.

Take the stairs You have heard this before, but climbing stairs is great exercise and easy to fit into your day when you've got the choice between a few flights and a lift. Fast, slow, skipping a stair in between, it's all good. Think of it as a little fitness bonus in your day every time you make this choice.

Take the hill If there is a choice between a flat route and a hilly one, take the time to walk, ride, or run up the hill once in a while. You don't have to be fast and the hill doesn't have to be very steep. Even a gradual incline will work different muscles and challenge you in a way that you'll notice. The cool thing about this is that you usually feel a little stronger in your next regular (non-hilly) workout, especially if you tackle a hill as a regular part of your routine.

Everything counts Look for ways to incorporate more activity into your day. Park further away from your office entrance, take your dog for a longer walk, spend 20 minutes working in your garden or cleaning your house, throw a ball or go for a bike ride with your kids, meet a friend for a walk instead of sitting down at a table, do some stretching or weight work while you watch TV. You get the idea, and you'll be surprised how naturally some of these things can fit in to your life.

Rest and recovery

People often misunderstand the concept of recovery. Minor aches or soreness in your muscles after a workout are not necessarily bad. Take it easier when you experience this, but, generally, gentle movement will help you recover better from this kind of soreness than doing nothing. If your legs ache after a run, take a walk or a yoga class the next day rather than avoiding movement altogether. To minimise soreness, make sure you take a few minutes to warm up (see page 144) before you work out; don't skip over that part when you look at your Programme plan.

During a hard workout, you need to rest and recover for a minute or more between tough efforts, exercises or reps. After you work out, take time to stretch and/or strengthen your muscles, depending on what type of workout you did. Refuel with protein and carbohydrates, and drink water to rehydrate adequately. You should also alternate the types of training you do so that different muscles and systems in your body have a chance to rest, repair and recover between workouts. This is when your body is really building and improving. The workouts on The Programme are designed to help you find this balance.

Finally, your workouts will be most effective when you listen to your body. They should never be painful or make you sick. If you feel nauseous, dizzy, breathless or faint while you're exercising: stop. The same goes if you experience pain in your chest, arms, neck or jaw: stop. A good workout should make you feel the muscles you are working, and allows time for recovery.

BONUS WORKOUT: STRETCH YOURSELF

Flexibility training is often overshadowed by cardiovascular and strength training, but if you want to train hard without injury, you need to incorporate flexibility training into your workouts. Sometimes people are confused about whether to stretch before or after working out, and this, plus impatience and time constraints, leads some to skip stretching altogether. That is a mistake. Please take my word for it, and don't wait for your body to let you know! The ideal time to work on flexibility training is right after you exercise, and it doesn't have to take a long time.

The key to proper stretching lies in the way you perform the stretch. When you're stretching certain parts of your body correctly, you should not feel pain. Staying relaxed is very important to stretching properly, and deep, easy, even breathing is the key to relaxation. If you notice yourself holding your breath while you are stretching, stop and start again. Your shoulders, hands, and feet should all be kept relaxed as you stretch. Make sure your body is not tight. Perform each stretch slowly and evenly. Hold the stretch for about 15 seconds and release slowly. Never bounce or jerk while stretching. This can cause injury if your muscle is pushed beyond its ability. All stretches should be smooth and slow. Flexibility exercises should be relaxing. Go slow and try to enjoy it.

Current guidelines from the American College of Sports Medicine recommend that stretching exercises for the major muscle groups be performed two or three times per week. Here are some basic stretches you should incorporate into your fitness programme, whenever it is convenient for you.

HAMSTRINGS

Set-up: Stand with your feet shoulder-width apart, extend your right leg straight in front of you and bend your left knee.

Action: Keep your back long and lean forward from the hips over the straight leg. Make sure not to lock out the right knee, keep it slightly bent. Your hands should rest on your bent knee. Stop when you feel a pull in the hamstring. Hold for 30 seconds. Repeat with the other leg.

QUADRICEPS

Set-up: Stand on your right foot and grasp your left foot.

Action: Tuck your pelvis in and gently pull your heel to your glutes. Hold for 30 seconds. Repeat with the other leg. *Use a sturdy chair or table if you need help balancing.*

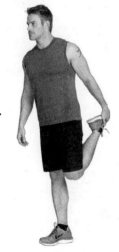

GLUTES AND HIPS

Set-up: Lie on your back, with legs extended. Bend your right knee and place your left ankle on your right thigh.

Action: With both hands, gently pull the bent knee towards your chest. Hold for 30 seconds. Repeat with the other leg.

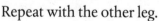

CHEST OPENERS

Set-up: Stand with your arms crossed at chest level.

Action: Stretch your arms out and back, feeling your chest and shoulders open. Hold for two breaths.

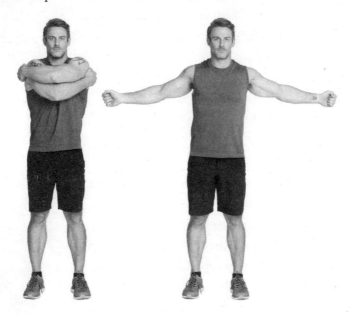

Sleep

It almost goes without saying that you will perform your best when you are well rested. The problems associated with being chronically overtired are both mental and physical, and will affect your appetite, your hormones, your stress level and the way your body processes food. Most adults need seven to eight hours of sleep a night. If you have trouble getting enough sleep, make it a priority to improve.

It helps to wake up and go to bed at a consistent time every day, which depends on your schedule and, optimally, your own body rhythms. Try making your bedroom relatively cool, as lightproof as possible, and don't have any screens (for example,

TV, computers, phones) in there if you can help it. If that's unavoidable, try limiting your use of them before bedtime, preferably shutting everything down at least an hour or two before you go to sleep. Once you start moving more, you will very likely sleep better. And when you are getting adequate sleep, you'll really notice a difference when you work out.

PRACTICAL DETAILS

Plan ahead

We make time for the things that are important. Giving yourself the gift of health is very important. Prioritise it. After the four-day Cleanse, you'll need to find about 45 minutes in your day – every day – to devote to exercise. These minutes do not need to be consecutive, but they do need to be planned for. I know it's appealing to see a fitness programme that promises big changes from only 10 minutes a day. This is not that. While little things add up and some movement is better than no movement, if you want to see significant results, you need to make a significant effort. So get out your calendar and schedule your time. For some of you, that might mean setting the alarm clock 30 minutes earlier. For others, it might mean spending your lunch hour differently a few times a week, or you may need to work out a childcare swap with a friend. Whatever it is you need to do to facilitate the time for exercise, it's worth it. You may even start to look forward to it.

There are certain exercises you can do while you're multitasking, even watching TV. Sometimes it helps to break up your workouts into smaller chunks during the day. You may need to switch your exercise timeframe on different days of the week – most people do. Try different strategies until you find what works for you, then make it non-negotiable.

What to wear

If you are motivated by having new or special workout clothes, go ahead. But you really don't need to wear anything special to do these workouts: loose, comfortable, stretchy shirts, shorts or tracksuit bottoms are all fine. Some people prefer the feeling of a technical, sweat-wicking fabric to a cotton T-shirt, but the choice is yours. Do get a decent pair of trainers. Some of the exercises could be done barefoot, but I generally recommend that my clients wear supportive trainers for working out. Take a few minutes the evening before to get everything ready, so you can move right into your Wake Up workouts the next morning.

FITNESS TERMS

Sets and reps
You will see the terms 'sets' and 'reps' in the instructions for your Strength training workouts.

- a 'set' is a group of successive repetitions performed with no rest in between the exercises. You might be asked to do four different exercises in a set.
- a 'rep' is short for repetition: it's the number of times you repeat an exercise in each set. You might be asked to repeat a particular exercise five times (5 reps) before moving on to the next one in the set.

Example: If I ask you to do 3 sets of 12 reps of press-ups, you would do 12 press-ups (1st set), rest, then complete 12 more press-ups (2nd set), rest again, and finish with 12 more press-ups (3rd set). ➤

Interval training

Your Athletic training workouts and Metabolic training workouts give you a specific amount of time to perform the exercises and a specific amount of time to rest. This is high intensity interval training, and you are meant to really push yourself to get the correct number of reps done in time and then rest just enough to recover and do it again. This gets your heart rate up, boosts your metabolism and makes for a very effective use of your workout time.

One form of interval training is Tabata, which consists of 20 seconds of work and 10 seconds of rest, repeated for 4 minutes. The Programme workouts in these areas are designed to introduce you to this style of working out. They are challenging, but also brief. You can do it!

Cool down

The cool down simply means doing something easy like walking or stepping on the spot instead of abruptly stopping after exercise. Stopping exercising suddenly can cause dizziness. Spend a few minutes in gentle motion to let your heart rate return to normal. The blood vessels in your legs expand during strenuous exercise, which brings more blood to your legs and feet; if you stop exercising too suddenly, your heart rate slows quickly and that blood can pool in your lower body and cause you to feel dizzy or even faint. So don't just sit down when you complete your sets, take a few moments at the end of your workout to 'cool down'.

Equipment for the workouts

Ideally you will have a mat, some dumb-bells, a bench or a sturdy chair, resistance bands and a stability ball. This equipment will give you a mini home gym and allow you to progress to more challenging exercises. But you can start The Programme with only a mat and a pair of dumb-bells.

You can find all these items online or at sports shops. Check out used/secondhand retailers, as they often have great deals on all the equipment you'll need.

Resistance bands

Resistance bands are great because they are cheap, compact, lightweight, portable and versatile. You can easily take them with you when you travel or if you want to do a quick workout at the office.

They generally come in three or four different levels of resistance. Look for bands that come with the door anchor attachment. Choose the appropriate level of resistance for you – the exercises that use the bands can be used with any of them.

Yellow (light)   Green (heavy)

Red (medium)   Blue or black (extra heavy)

Note: these are the colours traditionally used for physiotherapy bands, but dedicated fitness bands can vary in colour and corresponding resistance levels, so do check before buying.

Stability ball
(Swiss ball, balance ball, stretch ball, physio ball)

It doesn't really matter what you call it, just as long as you use it! Stability balls provide a great upper-body workout, a lower-body workout, a challenging abdominal workout, and can assist your stretching. How many things improve your balance and posture merely by sitting on them? Because the stability ball is an unstable surface, you have to use all the stability muscles in your core just to balance. You can also use the stability ball as a weight bench. Stability balls are usually sold in three sizes; choose the appropriate one for your height.

Height

1.5m to 1.62m (4'11" to 5'4")	55cm ball
1.62m to 1.8m (5'4" to 5'11")	65cm ball
1.8m (5'11" or above)	75cm ball

If you are at the cut-off height, try both sizes to see which feels best.

Dumb-bells

Dumb-bells are usually sold in pairs, or you can purchase an all-in-one variety, such as PowerBlock, which has options from 2.5kg to 23kg (5–50lb). However, the all-in-one options are more expensive and may not be necessary, depending on your fitness level. To start out you just need one light pair of dumb-bells and a heavy pair. For most women, a pair of 2.5kg (5lb) and 5kg (11lb) weights will get you started; for men, a pair of 7kg (15lb) and 11kg (25lb) dumb-bells might be a good starting point. But try them before you buy them.

When you use weights for strength-building exercises, you want them to be heavy enough to challenge your muscles to burn. That means, in general, that you should be lifting enough weight so that you are struggling to finish the last repetition of each set. For example, if you are doing biceps curls (see page 178) with 5kg (11lb) dumb-bells and at the end of the first set of 12 reps you feel like you could do 5 more reps, try increasing the weight to 6–7kg (13–15lb) dumb-bells.

Weight benches or steps

You will be lying on the bench or step for some of the upper body exercises and using it for leg exercises (step-ups and jumps), so the higher your bench or step is, the more challenging the exercise will be. The bench or step should ideally be high enough that when you step on it your knee is at a 90-degree angle.

Focus on form

The most important thing to focus on during all your workouts is your form: the 'quality not quantity' of each exercise. Pay attention to this, especially at the beginning, and maybe do a practice few before starting the sets to make sure you understand the goal of the exercise. If you find, during the set, that you need to take a break or do fewer reps in order to maintain good form, do it, because that is always better than continuing the exercise with poor form.

SQUATS

Keep your chest open.

Keep your core tight.

Keep your back straight, with a neutral spine.

Lower to 90 degrees. If you don't complete the full range of motion, you are not fully engaging your glutes and hamstrings. Your weight should be on the heels and balls of your feet.

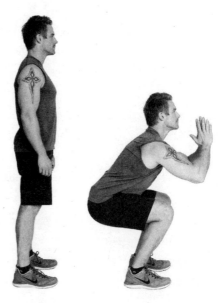

DEAD LIFT

Bend at your hip joint, not at your waist.

Look forward.

Don't round your back.

Keep dumb-bells close to your legs.

Squeeze your glutes to pull yourself up.

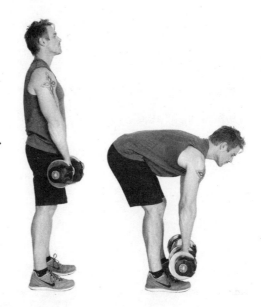

PRESS-UPS

Keep your head in a neutral position.

Place your hands straight on the floor beneath your shoulders, fingers pointed forward.

Keep elbows in (don't flare).

Push up, tighten your abs and squeeze your glutes.

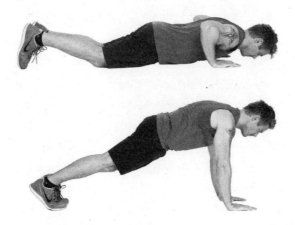

DUMB-BELL ROW

Keep your chest open.

Keep a straight line from the top of your head to your tailbone.

Tighten your abs.

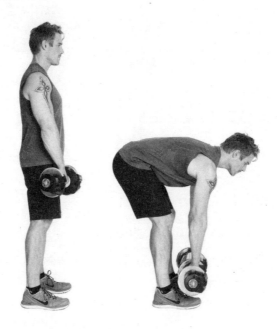

Set goals to get results

It's fine to want to be thinner, and it can be a motivating goal to get you to work out. But I think it helps to decide if you want to be fitter, stronger, healthier, more flexible and/or more agile, and to measure your progress in those terms in realistic ways. Having smaller goals – such as I want to be able to lift this much weight, or do this many reps of that exercise, or walk this many miles – will help you focus your attention and make the most of your physical training.

Take a breath!

We all know how to breathe, right? You're doing it right now, without even thinking about it, but when you exercise you need to think about how to breathe. We all have different instincts about breathing when we work out and most of them do not support an optimal performance. I've worked with people who hold their breath when they are doing high intensity workouts and others who are breathing quickly before they even warm up. Here are the breathing strategies you should follow during all your workouts:

Strength training Inhale on the less strenuous phase and exhale on the hardest part of the exercise. As an example, when you do a press-up, exhale as you push yourself up and inhale as you lower down.

Athletic/Metabolic high intensity training During high intensity training, your breath should come from the diaphragm, not the chest. That means that when the level of intensity ramps up, you should inhale through your nose and exhale through your mouth. These are demanding cardio workouts and they can leave you breathless, so be sure to take calm, deep breaths during the recovery intervals.

Slow-burn cardio During steady state cardio workouts your goal should be to maintain steady breathing in a comfortable manner. In other words, you should be able to have a conversation with someone while you are moving.

Flexibility Try to inhale and exhale in equal lengths, as slow deep breathing can increase your ability to go deeper into your stretches. Your nerves control the stretch reflex and when your body senses that a muscle is being stretched beyond its normal range of motion, your nerves will signal the muscles to contract in order to protect the muscles from damage. You can delay that stretch reflex by breathing deeply and exhaling into the stretch, and then you will be better able to hold the stretch longer. Try to maintain each stretch for 30–45 seconds. Remember not to stretch a cold muscle; this kind of stretching should be performed after your workouts, not before.

CHAPTER 5

THINK

....

Getting fit is not just about how you move and what you eat, but also how you think about your body. From the very beginning of The Programme, I emphasise that it's important to think about your 'why'. Staying focused will strengthen your commitment and increase your energy to succeed, and will also make it easier to keep on track if things feel like a grind. Identifying and understanding your why requires self-awareness, and there are practical things you can do to cultivate awareness in your life.

I believe that we all wake up every morning full of potential to be our best and make it a great day. Then we get busy. We spend our days zooming through our to-do lists, running from one task or obligation to another, taking care of others, and trying to fit everything in. This is the reality of most of our everyday lives. The problem is that when we don't make time to stop and pay attention to why and how we're doing all the things we do, we lose our sense of purpose and meaning and, often, our power. When that happens, many of us engage in behaviours that start to make us feel stuck, anxious and stressed out. We don't even realise what we're doing. Or maybe we can see ourselves doing things we know are unproductive but don't know how to stop. The Programme requires you to take time to pay attention to yourself, accept where you are, and figure out how to get where you need to be.

Hey, I know that there are a lot of people and things in your life worthy of your attention. But you're one of them. When you put everyone else's needs in front of your own – those of your kids, your spouse, your parents, your boss, your pet – no one gets the best of you. Many of my clients struggle with making time for this kind of self-care. It is not selfish to meet your own needs, and it will benefit everyone around you. Ultimately it means taking responsibility for yourself.

During The Programme, you are going to create a routine of healthy 'mind' rituals and see how you feel after practising them for one cycle. Everyone is different, so give each practice a chance and evaluate what worked best for you, what didn't, and why. Most people find some of these practices keep them focused on their eating and training goals. By the way, you don't have to be in any kind of distress to benefit from these practices. Think of them as tools in your toolbox to help you be a little happier. Or like secret weapons for getting fit and living well.

There are four ways you'll be harnessing your mind power during The Programme: set intentions, breathe, pay attention and be grateful. These don't have to take a lot of time, so I'm going to ask you to employ some form of all four of them every day.

SET INTENTIONS

If you have any experience of practising yoga, you may have come across the idea of setting an intention. I want you to set an intention for the day each morning. It can be a dedication, an attitude, a wish, a mission statement, an inspirational quote, a focal point, anything that sets the tone for how you want your day to unfold. Think of your intention as a seed, a kind of potential, that has the power to grow into something big as you cultivate and nurture it.

Intentions are not the same as goals, but they can help guide you towards your goals. Name your goals. They can – and should – be both large and small. Why are you doing The Programme? What do you want to change about your body or your life? What do you want to accomplish in the next week? In the next month? The next year?

Some people find this process really uncomfortable. Do it anyway. Don't be superstitious, afraid of failing, or be scared to say your goals out loud or write them down. Don't expect to achieve them overnight. My clients who are able to maintain weight loss and a healthy lifestyle understand that setting goals means you risk disappointing yourself, but also that you increase the possibility of learning from yourself and figuring out how to do better tomorrow. Once you have set some goals for yourself and are ready to start The Programme, take a minute or two each morning to set an intention for the day that helps you stay on track towards these goals.

Remember, this is not a to-do list, it's just a way to bring focus and meaning to the start of your day. You don't have to write it down, but I think it helps: you can add it as a note on your phone, send an email to yourself, write it out in a notebook dedicated to this practice, whatever works for you. Intentions are extremely personal. Examples of intentions people have shared with me include:

'I am going to get up and move today.'

'Today I'm going to say I can.'

'I am going to be brave today.'

'I am strong.'

'I am lovable.'

'I am loved.'

'I am good.'

'I am beautiful.'

'I'm going to go the extra mile today.'

'I am worth it.'

I want you to try this, even if it feels weird or awkward. It is a small thing that I have seen be a powerfully effective tool for keeping people on track when they are establishing new habits. There are other ways to do it: you might find inspiration for your daily intention in a photograph of a place or person you love, or that reminds you of somewhere that you want to be or a state of mind you want to experience. Visualising is a common training tool for athletes. They visualise themselves performing correctly over and over, and when they train, they visualise themselves getting stronger and reaching a specific goal. You can do this too. And it doesn't have to be only in your imagination. Having a picture of yourself that you like or of someone who inspires you or reminds you of where you want to be can be a good motivator. I have a client who uses images to set her intentions, and she will take a screen shot of something inspiring to look at and set it on the lock screen on her phone each day. Think about what motivates you or what you're excited about for the day and take a minute to set your intention.

Being conscious of your intentions is a crucial component of living well. It is so important to be positive, to focus on the healthy behaviours you are engaging in and the reasons that you're changing. Every day is a new day and another opportunity to do it better. Setting intentions helps you to remind yourself of that, and is even more important after those days when you make choices you regret. If you screwed up last night, move forward. Notice how you felt. You need to remember that feeling and use it to stay powerful in the new day when setting your new intention.

Going the extra mile If you find you have time in the morning, and enjoy the process of writing, you can expand on the intention and write in more detail about how you're feeling and what you're excited about. Don't feel pressured to do that; setting the intention is enough. But some people want to go deeper.

Vision boards also work for certain people. This is a bulletin board where you display images that represent where you want to be in any or all areas of your life. Think of it as a visual map of photographs, drawings, quotations, or anything else that inspires you and connects you with your dreams. Look at it purposefully in the morning or just have it around where your subconscious mind can take it in: visualising success can reinforce your intentions and your willpower.

BREATHE

So many things compete for our time, fragmenting our concentration. It's easy to become distracted and overwhelmed. Focusing on your breath is a quick and effective technique both for calming down and reminding yourself of your priorities, whatever they are. As you go through your day and take a bit of a beating here and there, eroding your goodwill and motivation, remember that you can shut your eyes, breathe deeply and not let everything simply happen to you.

Obviously you're breathing all the time without thinking about it. But as you start to reconnect with yourself as a physical being – rather than just living 'in your head' – you'll be paying more conscious attention to your breath. There are specific techniques you can use for breathing while you're working out, which I covered on page 109, but I'm talking about something different here.

Take a moment to stop during the day, especially if you find yourself feeling stressed, and focus on your breathing. You might be surprised at how often you discover yourself holding your breath. It's a subconscious way of attempting to control emotion and anxiety. If you notice that you're doing it, just take a long inhale and exhale, and repeat. You'll figure out what feels comfortable for you. If you're having trouble, I once heard someone describe this to a child in this way: 'Picture yourself holding a piece of hot pizza. Smell the pizza, then blow on the pizza.' The point is simply to take a moment to breathe very consciously.

As your mind wanders all over the place, which it inevitably will, try simply concentrating on your breath. You don't have to do this for a long time: you can take 10 or 20 deep breaths and think of yourself as recharging. This is a way of both keeping your power and, sometimes, tuning into important information about what's going on in your body.

Practices that have us tune in to our breath and calm down can help reduce stress and blood pressure, and strengthen the immune system. Most of us live in our heads more than our bodies and we don't tune in to ourselves physically: we pay no attention when things are going well and – either consciously or subconsciously – we use various strategies to block out painful physical sensations or emotions. But our bodies have so much to tell us about how we're doing, both physically and emotionally. When you deliberately pay attention to yours, starting with your breath, you'll be better able to see how particular things are affecting you.

Breathing consciously can help you detach from your emotions even as you tune in and notice them. Finally, breathing can also give us a really good clue to our state of mind. You might notice that it changes and calms while – and just because – you're paying attention to it. Think of paying attention to your breath as a quick way of shifting gears when you start to feel overwhelmed. You can do this in the car, at your desk, in the bathroom, literally any time you need to take a minute – it doesn't have to be on any kind of schedule and no one needs to know you're doing it.

Going the extra mile There are a lot of specific breathing techniques you can explore to use in different situations. One that many people find effective when they need to harness energy or focus is called alternate nostril breathing, which might sound strange, but is worth a try. When you're sitting comfortably, use your right thumb to press your right nostril closed and then inhale deeply in through your left nostril. At the peak of that inhale, use your right index finger to close off the left nostril, release your thumb and exhale through your right nostril. Repeat this pattern a few times, continuing to inhale through the left side of your nose and exhaling through the right side, and see if you don't feel more clear. This is only one of many simple, directed breathing exercises you can try. You'll find many others widely available online.

PAY ATTENTION

In addition to getting into the habit of paying attention to your breath in order to stay calm and tune into your body, you also need to cultivate the habit of paying attention to your thoughts. Starting The Programme means that you've set goals for yourself: to achieve those goals you need to harness your mind power. The messages we give ourselves every day are very powerful and yet we tend not to be mindful about them.

Being mindful means paying attention to things you wouldn't normally notice and I want you to get into the habit of setting aside some time each day to deliberately pay some calm attention to your own experience as it unfolds, without judgement. Tuning in to where you're at in the moment means taking a few minutes to be purposefully conscious of your mind and body. There are several ways to do this, and I want you to try them out as they fit your schedule. But try them all over the course of The Programme.

If you have 5 minutes today Stop whatever you are doing. Close the door, shut your phone off (or set a 5-minute timer on it), stop moving and withdraw. Close your eyes. Allow the cascade of thoughts in your mind to settle. This takes time and can feel uncomfortable. You are not sleeping or resting. Don't try to control what your mind is thinking. Just stay still and notice your feelings and experiences. Don't worry about why you're having particular thoughts or what to do about them, just notice them. Don't judge them. There is no right or wrong.

Do you notice any physical sensations in your body? Where are they? What are they like? Do you feel a particular emotion? How do you know you're experiencing it? Do you feel it physically? What thoughts are you having? Again, simply notice whatever comes to mind and then let it flow by, like a passing cloud. There is no need to try to analyse, understand, or change any of your observations, just notice them. When 5 minutes has passed, you can stop and move forward with your day.

If you have 15 minutes today Shut your phone off (or set a timer) and find a quiet space. You can sit on a chair or on the floor, lie down or stand up, in whatever position feels comfortable, but maybe not lying on your bed or the sofa, because you don't want to be so relaxed that you fall asleep. Get comfortable, close your eyes and take a few deep breaths. Don't try to filter any thoughts, noise or other sensations, simply notice them and try to focus on your breath. Some people find it helps to focus on their breath moving through a specific body part as they do this, either their nose, chest, belly or mouth. When your mind wanders, just notice the thought and then redirect your attention to the in and out of your breathing.

Other people find visualising an image helps them stay focused on the breath. Imagine a small light in the centre of your breastbone. As you inhale, imagine that light expanding. As you exhale, imagine the light receding back to its original small size. When your mind wanders, you can bring it back to the breath and the image of the light.

No time? If you are thinking, 'Jessie, you've got to be kidding – I have no extra time today,' you are not off the hook! Another way of practising mindfulness is by observing yourself doing a small task. So try really paying attention to something you might normally do unconsciously. The classic example is washing the dishes; another one I think is useful is folding the laundry. Instead of multitasking and watching TV or talking on your phone while you fold the laundry, try really giving this chore your full attention and notice all your senses and bodily sensations as you experience it. What do the clean clothes smell like? How do the different fabrics and textures feel in your hands? How are you feeling as you fold? Are you hunching your shoulders? In other words, give this chore your complete attention. As with the other mindful practices, try not to judge or change any of these thoughts, just be with them. Alternatively, you can try doing this when you brush your teeth – I know you're fitting that in, or at least I hope you are.

You might be wondering how this all this fits into your physical fitness goals. In addition to its other benefits, being mindful in this meditative way helps you practise discipline and willpower. When I am doing these types of exercises, I often find myself thinking about things I need to do. I remember obligations that feel urgent, like an email I forgot to respond to or a call I promised to make. Those tasks are real and I have to do them, or at least write them down so I don't forget about them. But in that moment that I am thinking about them instead I wait, because I have made a decision to make space for mindfulness, so whatever I'm remembering has to keep for 15 minutes. Every time I do this it gets easier. Now, there may be times when you feel an urgent need to snack or eat, or an impulse to mindlessly eat food at work or at a party when you aren't actually hungry. Once you have established a habit of pausing for a few minutes in one area, you may find it easier to pause in this other area, to stop and say OK, I notice that impulse, let me get back to it in 5 or 10 minutes. You're breaking the habit of needing to act on your impulses immediately and being mindful about the action you are about to take. Essentially, you are treating your thoughts like thoughts – not like instructions that must be followed or absolute truths you must believe.

Going the extra mile We have explored some simple meditative exercises, but there are many ways to take the practice of meditation further. Some of them can be physical, like yoga, t'ai chi or qi gong, and certain kinds of dance. There are other ways of meditating that are totally stationary. There are silent styles of meditation and others that involve chanting, candles, music or someone else guiding you with words. These all 'work', but some might be more comfortable for you than others. If you're interested, you can explore other types of meditation practices, either through what's available in your community or through books in your local library. There are also some meditation resources available online, including on my website Pavelka.co.uk: feel free to use it to explore what is most effective for you.

BE GRATEFUL

At night, we tend to think we had a 'good day' or a 'bad day' – and that's if we haven't already moved on to our list of things we need to get done tomorrow. The truth is that you had many different moments and experiences today. Take a minute at the end of the day and pick three things that made you happy or that you can feel grateful for. Write them down in a notebook or a file on your computer or phone dedicated to this purpose. You are going to do this throughout The Programme. Some days it will be easy, other days you might have to dig a little, but it shouldn't take you more than a minute or two, and I guarantee that if you think about it you will find at least three moments to be grateful for each night.

What you write should be specific but does not need to be detailed. It could be a major milestone or a fleeting moment. Some examples of things people have shared with me from their gratitude lists include:

'Hydrangeas blooming today.'

'Ate a perfect peach.'

'Taking my kids to swings at the park.'

'Walked after dinner.'

'Loving new book that I started today.'

'Email from my son.'

'Saw amazing sunrise when walking the dog.'

'Did record number of press-ups in 60 seconds.'

'My hair looked really good.'

'Made it to the gym after all.'

You get the idea. You're stopping to be aware of what went right today, and it's OK if those things were small. This will help you to be conscious of the things you have to be grateful for, the things that bring you satisfaction, and the things that engage and inspire you.

This is not a journal or diary. The contents of your list will help you to notice patterns when you have been doing this for a little while. If you see that going for a walk after dinner makes you happy, or that getting up early enough to see the sun rise was on your list three times over a couple of weeks, maybe you should try to do those things more often. Many people are sur-prised at how often movement-based activity turns out to be a high point of their day, and recording it encourages them to do it more often. Whatever it is that's making you happy, keep doing it.

The other great thing about recording the things that make you happy is that you can flip back when you're feeling low or discouraged, and see how much you have to be grateful for when you look at the 'big picture'. Many people find it satis-fying to look at their lists as they get longer, it helps them get per-spective and celebrate the good stuff. Also, you might find that the habit of doing this makes you more tuned in to those moments when they are actually happening. Notice what they feel like. You don't have to try to create them. They are already happening to you.

HARNESSING YOUR MIND POWER

All four of the 'think' practices I've asked you to try can be done in 5 minutes or less. While you can benefit from spending more time on some of them, you don't have to, and the potential payoff for less than 20 minutes a day is tremendous. You may experience some relaxation or have an important insight during some of these exercises. If you do, that's great, but don't feel like these are goal oriented – there's no failing. And there's rarely an ultimate victory: there will probably not be a moment where you say to yourself, I'm amazing, I'm conscious, grateful, and totally in tune with the universe (if you have one, let me know how you did it!). The goal of these exercises is to help you become more in tune with yourself, and to use that knowledge to help your physical training and self-discipline in several ways.

As you pay attention to your thoughts, you can eventually redirect the unproductive ones and change your experience. When you are actively slowing down to do these exercises, don't judge your thoughts or respond to them, just notice them and let them pass. But pay attention. Are some of your thoughts repetitive? defeating? negative? distracting? Many of us find it so uncomfortable to have those kinds of thoughts that we do unhelpful things – such as unnecessary eating or drinking – to avoid them. You'll be developing the discipline to simply sit with those kinds of feelings.

Many people who have struggled with their weight or fitness have self-defeating thoughts about their ability to become healthier. If you are nervous about whether you can be successful, these 'Think' exercises can help you get comfortable with accepting the idea of failure. If you're scared, accept it. You might fail. It's a possibility. A lot of trainers will tell you when you think you can't do something, that you need to change your attitude; that if you accept failure as a possibility, you will fail. This is kind of a 'refuse to lose' mentality. I'm going to go ahead and say 'Transformation is scary, yes, you might fail. Acknowledge it, accept it, and decide you want to go for it anyway and see what happens.' The practice of actively noticing your feelings teaches you not to resist anxious or uncomfortable feelings. Just accept that you have them and let them exist while you take action. This is more of a 'feel the fear and do it anyway' philosophy.

Everything you need to be successful exists inside you right now. When you use discipline to build strength and clarity in your mind, you are moving towards feeling better in your body. When you use your mind power to stick to actions that bring you closer to your intentions, you will be more free to grow, you will feel in control and be happier. That possibility is worth 20 minutes of your day.

CHAPTER 6

CONNECT

Your success in reaching your goals depends on you taking responsibility for your own health and fitness. But you don't have to do it alone, and you shouldn't. The quality of your relationships affects your happiness and well-being, your motivation and performance, and your accountability and health. Taking some time to pay attention to four key relationships, and cultivate some healthy ones, is part of The Programme.

The Connect practices are different from your 'Think' exercises. I don't expect you to set aside specific time for all four of your major relationship areas every day, although you'll need an accountability partner that you check in with pretty regularly. However, after reviewing this section, I'd like you to commit to taking one action each day to enhance one of these relationships and to work on connecting in all four of these areas of your life for the duration of The Programme – and beyond.

CONNECT WITH YOURSELF

Let's start with an important relationship that most people overlook: the one you have with yourself. When you do some of the exercises in the Think section of The Programme, you'll be starting to tune in to your experience, both physical and emotional. The practice I want you to try here is somewhat different, because rather than just acknowledging your feelings and getting comfortable with the tough ones, you're going to take some action to challenge them, in order to connect – or reconnect – with your best self.

Our thoughts dictate our moods. Everything starts with a thought. When you pay attention to the thought patterns that you are allowing to run through your head, it will give you some insight into what makes you feel a certain way. So, if you can redirect the negative thoughts, it may help you to become a stronger, more self-loving person.

Change the thought pattern – change the feeling. It really is that simple. If you don't like what you are watching on the TV or listening to on the radio, what do you do? You change the channel, right? You can learn to do the same with your thought patterns.

Look at yourself. And listen

Set some time aside when you can be alone and look at yourself in a mirror. A full-length mirror is ideal, but a smaller one is OK. Really look into your own eyes, look at your face and body and think about where you have been and what you want for yourself. Stay still and look for longer than you want to, maybe five full minutes. Most people find this to be a very weird and uncomfortable experience, but it's important. I find that it generally triggers challenging and helpful insights.

You might not like what you see. That's OK. Tell yourself this is Day 1 and keep looking. I worked with a client, Sara, who did the exercise with me in the room. I asked her what she saw in the mirror and she said, 'I hate myself.'

I told Sara that nothing was going to change until she started loving herself, and I asked her to think of some good things about herself. You should do this too, if you're not already doing it naturally. If you find it difficult to identify things about your physical being that you can feel good about, focus on your experience as a person. Think about things you may have overcome or endured, experiences that made you feel powerful and strong. I have worked with people who were in very low places, emotionally and physically. Someone cast around for something good to say about himself until he came up with, 'I guess I'm still here.'

If that's where you are, hold on to that thing, whatever it is that gives you a bit of power. It can be something about your body, such as liking your smile or your eyes; it can be a memory of a physical triumph, like running a race or giving birth to your child; it can be the knowledge that you've endured something painful and are still here, like the loss of a job or the death of a family member. The point is that you are re-establishing a relationship with yourself that needs to be honest and kind, in the same way that you hope your best relationships with other people would be. You may need to change the conversation with yourself. To that end, notice the way you observe yourself and try reframing some of your negative observations:

'My legs are too big' can become 'My legs are strong.'

'My arms are sore' can become 'My arms are changing and getting stronger.'

'I've got a long way to go' can become 'I'm worth the struggle.'

You get the idea. If it helps, think about what you would say if you heard a friend you cared about say something self-defeating. You would, hopefully, be honest in your response but also encouraging and optimistic. Show yourself the same care and repeat this exercise with the mirror once a week throughout The Programme.

Know your negatives

The catalyst for many of my clients is feelings of self-loathing. They just can't stand to look – or live – a particular way any longer. But that presents a problem: it might get you started, but you won't sustain your changes without changing your outlook.

We all have facets of ourselves that we feel self-conscious or unhappy about. You don't want those negative thoughts to transform into destructive behaviour patterns that make you feel out of control. Sometimes I ask people to give themselves 10 minutes on the clock – no longer – to write down all the negative thoughts that they are struggling with, even if they seem crazy. When the time is up, take a deep breath, review your list and respond to it in a rational, positive way. Try to reframe your fear as excitement and see the opportunities in the obstacles you face. Try to focus on the things your body can do as opposed to the parts of it you want to change.

Remember – or rediscover – what makes you happy

Many clients who start The Programme find that moving more makes them happy. The actual time in the gym may be painful – although more people than you'd expect really look forward to some parts of their workout – but almost everyone finds that post-exercise feeling to be a source of pleasure. For some, this is a brand new discovery, for others, it's a reminder of a feeling they had as a student or just a kid running around.

What other experiences, either in your past or in your dreams, do you want to explore? I think that in the same way that we all have bodies that are designed to move, we all have a creative instinct that can bring us pleasure and happiness if we can tap into it. My dad plays in a band and I grew up surrounded by music, but I didn't pick up an instrument until I was twenty-five, when I taught myself to play the guitar. Now, I'm not ready to go out in public with it, but I find playing and writing music to be a really satisfying outlet. It makes me feel good when I'm sad and it allows me to use my brain and body in ways that are completely different from how I spend most of my working days.

Do you have a creative outlet like this? Don't think about it too much, just consider something that excites you, and tap into the process. You can reconnect with a skill or interest that you have – or try something that's completely new. I have clients who paint, draw, make music, knit, sew, cook or carve. And you don't have to have any kind of agenda or improvement plan in this area. This is about the process, not the end result: if you try, for example, drawing with a pencil and paper for an hour one night this week instead of watching TV, whatever you wind up with is entirely beside the point. The goal is just to immerse yourself, however briefly, in the meditative process of creating something.

Don't just dream about your creativity, take action. Write down three things you liked to do when you were a kid. Let's say you liked reading, riding your bike and colouring-in. Do them this week. Alternatively, think about three things you've always wanted to learn how to do. Maybe that's painting, playing an instrument or learning another language. Pick one and make a plan to try it out.

Doing small things differently

Another way of reconnecting with yourself is by shaking up your routine in small ways. I know The Programme may require you to make larger changes in the way you eat and schedule movement into your day. Be open to experiencing other aspects of your life differently as well. Take a different route to work. Work out at different times of the day and night. Make one meal of foods that are entirely new to you. Go to a street or a local area you've never been to before. You get the idea: these changes don't have to be a big deal. But doing things a little differently will make you more conscious of the things around you. Think about when you drive a route that you've never taken before compared with one you are very familiar with. You're more alert and watchful, usually, if you have to take a new path. Cultivate this quality of wakefulness in your life in general.

CONNECT WITH A HIGHER POWER

We all have moments when life seems overwhelming. For some of my clients, overeating has been a way of getting through the day. When you are struggling to believe in your own ability to take care of yourself, having a belief in something outside of yourself, something higher than yourself, can be a useful way of confronting the tough moments, keeping things in perspective, and making better choices.

It can be helpful if there is something or someone that you feel you can hand your stress and anxiety over to. I grew up in a religious home and have seen the great things that faith can do for people. Some of my clients have found religious faith to be a significant source of strength, inspiration and support as they struggle to make changes in their lives. Everyone's relationship to their faith is different, but one thing I've noticed is that worship services tend to have moments of complete stillness that are rare in most of our lives. We don't generally make much room for silence, reflection and time for just 'being' instead of 'doing'.

You don't have to be a practising member of a particular religion to have those moments. As a boy, I played outside all day long and I continue to feel very connected to something greater than me – nature. I think being outside, especially early in the morning in a beautiful place, can help remind us that we are all a part of something much larger than ourselves. However you want to conceptualise it, looking up and out, being still, being present to what surrounds you, and making some space for wonder and reflection, will almost surely help you put your problems into a manageable perspective.

I recently climbed Snowdon in Wales with a group of people. It was one of the most spiritually enjoyable days I have experienced in a while. The scenery was outstanding and it got more amazing the higher we got. The air was thick and misty at the top of the mountain and I took a few minutes to slip away from the party and sit by myself and enjoy that view. I felt as though my heart was expanding as I breathed in the cool mountain air and allowed time to stand still. It felt like a moment of surrender. I felt connected, renewed and invigorated.

I encourage you to connect with something that has meaning for you. We are all different, and what a higher power means to each of us may vary. Yours could be music, art or the family environment. There are no hard and fast rules here. Whatever it is, give yourself up to it and allow that connection to fill your heart, support you and bring you peace.

During the Programme, make an effort to remind yourself that you are not alone. Get outside. Consider ways of exploring your own beliefs and strengthening your ties to whatever gives you comfort, and makes you feel elevated, calm, supported and connected to something greater than yourself.

CONNECT WITH FRIENDS AND ACCOUNTABILITY PARTNERS

When you are healthier and feeling good, you are going to have more energy and self-confidence, and this often translates into healthier relationships with other people in your life. While you are getting there, you need people, preferably a network of people, who can support you while you pursue your goals.

At an absolute minimum, you need one person who can serve as an accountability partner. This is a person with whom you can be honest about your goals, to whom you can be vulnerable, who understands what you want and can help you get there. In an ideal world, this is a person you can train with, who can encourage you and maybe who you can encourage as well. Your accountability partner may be someone who is in a similar position to you and can relate to your struggle, or it may be someone who is in outstanding and inspirational shape. The type of person who works best varies for each individual. Think about what you need most. Will it be support in the gym? Will it be emotional support? Identify a person who you can trust to be reasonably available for you to check in with, who will help you through this process.

Sometimes people have a hard time visualising their family members serving as accountability partners or being sources of support. If this applies to you, I encourage you not to write anyone off, because people can surprise you, and it's a big help when your partner and family get on board. But if yours won't, or they're far away, or just not going to be able to fulfil this function for you, know that family comes in many different forms, and support for a healthy lifestyle doesn't have to come from your blood relatives. You can connect to a network of people who are doing what you're doing and can encourage you. I have that at my gym; it's a place for me to connect with people as well as train, and it has a kind of family feeling for me. Most communities have resources of this kind and they don't have to be expensive. Look into gyms, including your local YMCA, cycling, walking and running groups and events, organised weight loss-groups, boot camps, yoga classes or fitness equipment: identify potentially appealing places for you to connect with other people who are doing what you're doing.

You also have online options for making fitness connections, including mine! Now that you've bought this book, you are part of The Programme family. The Pavelka House is an online resource that provides a wealth of information and inspiration to keep you motivated and updated, as well as being a great platform for linking up with other like-minded people. When I helped to design it, I wanted to create something that enhanced people's lives and helped keep them accountable, but didn't become a second job to keep it updated. I called it the House because it's somewhere you can check in to and feel part of something on your own terms.

The House is there when you need motivation or when you want to get ideas, record progress or celebrate with friends. People can have their own personal room in the House, too. Like any room, you can decorate it when you move in. It's a place to keep pictures that make you feel inspired. No one else sees your room, so you can be as personal as you like. If you like a particular recipe, workout exercise, motivational quote, or story, you can click and save it to your room, then take it out again when you're ready to move on.

Community is an important part of The Programme, and the forums and ability to comment on all of the articles in the House create conversation and interest among members, who learn from and encourage each other. One of my favourite parts of the House is the section where you can upload the events that you have set yourself as challenges. If you enter a 5K or a triathlon, you can upload the details, and others who are in the area can get in touch and compare notes or meet up with you for training or the event itself. It's great fun, and I love seeing the public pictures members upload afterwards!

The House is used differently by everyone. Some dip in and out for recipe ideas and workout suggestions, and maybe pop into the forums. Others are on there each day, and it has become part of their daily Programme planning. The journal function means that you can capture your progress, feelings and ideas. You are also able to set your monthly goals, and you will receive an email checking in with you each month so that you are reminded to update or change them.

All of these functions help you to stay on track with The Programme after reading the book, and I hope you'll check it out (you can connect through JessiePavelka.com.) Online accountability partners can be very effective. I have clients who check in daily by text or email with people they've never met, but a 'Did you work out today?' or 'How are things going?' message keeps them motivated. Responsible online forums and communities can also be good resources for information about exercise and nutrition. These are helpful for anyone, and sometimes they are your only option for geographic or logistical reasons. But if you find that you are limiting yourself to online support because you are too intimidated to walk into a physical gym or connect with people in person, I encourage you to make doing that one of your goals as you get more comfortable following The Programme. There are a lot of benefits to exercising with a partner or a group, which you can read about in more detail in the 'Sweat' section of this book. Connecting with others is one of them.

By the way, kids can be great at making you accountable. If you've promised to take them somewhere (swimming, to the park or any physical activity) they will not let you off the hook.

Trust me, I know this: my six-year-old certainly keeps me on my toes. If you share your fitness goals or commitments with your kids, you might find that they are relentless in keeping you accountable and, possibly, thrilled to join you in some of your activities. You know yours best.

One other thing about connecting with others: in the same way that I want you to pay some mind to how you are thinking about and talking to yourself, pay attention to the quality of your communication with your family and friends. Take a minute to be conscious of your patterns when you interact. Do you look at one another? Is anyone checking the phone or multi-tasking while you're together? Are you checking your email when you're speaking on the phone? Are people listening or interrupting each other? Is your mind wandering when the other person is talking? I'm not judging, and you shouldn't either. Every conversation we have isn't going to be a meaningful and reflective one. But notice what has become normal for you, and think about making an effort to improve the quality of the connections you have with the people you care about.

CONNECT WITH THE WIDER WORLD

I've noticed that unhappy clients often tend to withdraw from the world. It's understandable that when we don't feel good about ourselves, it's harder to feel positive or interested in engaging with others. I worked with a young guy, Ben, who had been overweight all his life and had experienced bullying and teasing as a boy to the extent that he simply assumed everyone was judging him negatively. As an adult he withdrew as a way of protecting himself and he had become socially isolated. Now, you may not be in such an extreme situation, but you might be unhappy with how you look, less socially confident than you wish you were, or maybe even just lonely. If this is you,

I understand the impulse to isolate when you are unhappy – but I know that it only intensifies and prolongs your suffering. The worse you feel, whether it's about your weight or something else, the more important it is for you to be connected with people who care about you and the wider world.

When you are considering who to choose as an accountability partner, as well as considering your immediate network of people, think beyond it and you may also be able to see various sources of potential support. Maybe there's one person who will work out with you on a more casual basis. Maybe there is someone else who can help you make time to fit exercise into your life, like a colleague who might be interested in walking together on your lunch break or a friend who might be willing to watch your kids for an hour while you work out. Is there someone who might share an interest in healthy food and cooking? How about people who care about you and can simply listen when you're frustrated, or celebrate your success? Every kind of support you are able to harness is going to help you, and you may find that your decisions inspire and support other people to make healthy changes in their lives as well. You just need to be brave enough to put your goals out there and enlist that help.

If you don't think you have those people, I am challenging you to find them by engaging in your community. Take a fitness class, sign up for an event, consider volunteering; anything that can expand your network to include other people who are also making healthy choices, and can help you stay motivated, encouraged and inspired. There is power in groups, in healthy competition, and in being stimulated by new experiences. Tapping into any of that will enhance your experience on The Programme.

I have noticed a really cool thing happening with a group of my clients. I always encourage people to set individual challenges, such as running a 5K race, to get them excited about their new way of life and give them something to aim for. What is happening more and more is that groups of my clients are coming together to train, practise and take part in a variety of different events and occasions. Mud runs, zip wires, spa weekends, charity runs, you name it: they are constantly surprising me with the ways they are finding to unite as a community through fitness. Their enthusiasm and energy is inspiring. Look for ways that you can bring people together. You don't have to wait for someone else to organise something, you can be a leader – a pioneer. You will bring joy and health to others and feel amazing.

A word about problem people

Some of my clients discover that one or more people they are connected with are not so supportive of their efforts to be healthy. It's very common and you do need to deal with it. If you notice that your partner keeps bringing home your favourite treats from the bakery or throws up obstacles when you are scheduling your workouts, or that your mother gets offended if you don't come back for seconds at her dinner table, try to talk to those people in a calm, non-judgemental way about what's happening: 'I'm noticing [this] and it makes it hard for me to do [that.]' See what they say. Sometimes well-meaning people don't understand your goals, or didn't realise how their behaviour is interfering with your efforts to get healthy. Other times, it's more complicated. If you find that there are people in your life who behave in a way – or have an opinion – that interferes with your path to better health, you need to set some boundaries.

Setting healthy boundaries doesn't mean cutting off a relationship. But if you are attached to people who make it hard for you to stick with The Programme, you need to sort out ways to interact with them that don't involve unhealthy food, don't interfere with your exercise, and don't make you feel bad about yourself. Sometimes this is as simple as suggesting meeting up with a friend over a coffee or morning walk instead of dinner or evening drinks at a bar. Sometimes it's more complicated, and disappointing, to discover that someone you want to rely on is not going to be able to support you in this way. Developing, and maintaining, a wider network of healthy relationships will go a long way towards helping you navigate this.

WORKING ON RELATIONSHIPS

The stronger all of these relationships in your life are, the better you're going to feel, and the more likely you are to achieve success on The Programme, however you define it. Cultivating these connections will take time, patience and some trial and error. Make it a priority to take one action each day to connect via one of these relationships. Put it on your to-do list if you have to, and notice if you tend to be cultivating one or two relationships at the expense of others. Try to spread your energy around. Plant seeds in all four areas over the course of each week, and look forward to seeing what blooms.

The Rest of Your Life

· ·

C hanging your body is also about changing your mind. There are many different ways to get results in a mirror or on the scales, but the key to living well over the long term is developing the ability to love and take care of yourself no matter what else is happening in your life. I hope that you'll use The Programme to eat, sweat, think and connect your way to the very best version of yourself.

Once you complete the first cycle of The Programme, take some time to reflect. Repeat the fitness assessments and evaluate your progress. Appreciate your amazing body and what it can do. Identify what parts of The Programme are going well and what is still challenging. Troubleshoot those challenges. Is your goal realistic? Are you making it a priority? Have you learned or improved anything during the process of chasing it, even if you have not reached it yet?

Be realistic. There are parts of your body that can be changed and others that are part of your genetic make-up. Understand the difference between them and don't waste time agonising about stuff that isn't in your control. Look at all the different types of athletic body shapes, notice how different they are, and how few of them are what we might call skinny. Seek out body images and messages that reinforce the power of good performance. You can control a lot: be consistent about your workouts, give them your all and fuel them properly. Don't only notice how you look. Notice how you feel.

I don't know you and I don't know what your goals are. But I hope, at this point in The Programme, that they aren't just about getting thin or skinny. Our bodies come in all shapes and sizes. Being strong is sexy. Being fit is powerful. Being confident is beautiful. Living well is inspiring. Being healthy frees up energy in your life to pursue the things and relationships that make you feel good. You can be all those things and look amazing and not be skinny. I hope you are thinking about yourself as an athlete, and that you understand the power that nutrition, rest and commitment have on your ability to perform at your best. I hope that you are becoming more aware of your unique gifts and potential, and are making richer connections with others that help support you in reaching your goals and enhancing your life.

You may be humbled and challenged at points on The Programme but I hope you're also getting to feel fully present and alive, and experiencing the satisfaction that comes from taking good care of yourself and pushing to be your very best. That may be stronger, slimmer and sexier, but fundamentally it's about living well.

The Workout Programme and Recipes

TRAINING SCHEDULE

Day	Programme
1	Strength assessment
2	Athletic assessment
3	Metabolic assessment
4	Slow Burn and Flow assessment
5	Metabolic training
6	Strength training
7	Athletic training
8	Strength training
9	Metabolic training
10	Strength training
11	Athletic training
12	Strength training
13	Slow Burn and Flow
14	Strength training
15	Athletic training
16	Strength training
17	Metabolic training
18	Strength training
19	Athletic training
20	Strength training
21	Metabolic training
22	Choose your training
23	Re-test starts
Extras	Weekend Warrior
	Yoga

CHAPTER 7

The Programme
WORKOUTS

....

The Programme is a 21-day cycle designed to get you started on the journey to lifelong fitness. In other parts of this book we have seen how eating well, taking time to move more, living mindfully and connecting with other people are the four essential elements of genuine fitness. This section shows you exactly how I want you to move your body on these 21 days.

It begins with four days of fitness assessments, which will determine the level at which you should start your training schedule. Each assessment should take you less than 20 minutes, including time sorting out the exercises. Review the moves and maybe do a practice one or two to make sure you've got it. Then, using a stopwatch, wristwatch or a phone with a timer, perform each one 'on the clock', and record the results.

I have divided the Programme workouts by level: Beginner, Intermediate and Advanced. As with all other areas of The Programme, I want this to be as flexible as possible so that it works for you. If you need to follow the Beginner exercises for the Strength workouts but are ready to do Intermediate for your

Athletic (agility) workouts, that's fine. Also, I want you to be able to use these workout plans for as long as possible. If you're improving when you repeat the assessment tests, take it to the next level workout and see how it feels.

Once you have completed the four assessment days, The Programme alternates days of 'Burn' and 'Build' workouts. Burn training is designed to improve your endurance (stamina) and agility, while the Build days work on building your strength. On both Burn and Build days, you will also do a Wake Up workout (see pages 168, 191 and 217).

DON'T SKIP THE WARM UP!

Whenever you are exercising, it's helpful to prime the body for movement. Spend about a minute doing each of the following movements before you get started with *any* of the workouts and assessments on The Programme. You don't have to worry about levels here, everyone can warm up in the same way. Repeat each exercise for 30–45 seconds.

SQUATS
Set-up: Stand with your feet hip-width apart, arms at your sides.
Action: Bend your knees, as if you're sitting on a chair, until your thighs are nearly parallel. Slowly return to the start position.

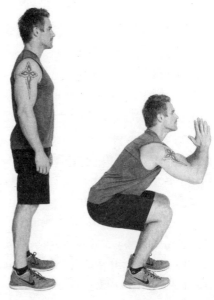

ARM CIRCLES

Set-up: Stand with your feet shoulder-width apart, arms at your sides.
Action: Slowly start to make circles with your arms fully extended. Continue ten times, then change direction.

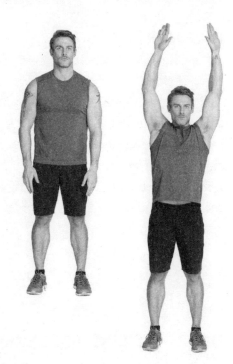

HIP OPENERS

Set-up: Stand with your feet hip-width apart.
Action: Raise your right knee up towards your chest and rotate it to the right in a circular motion, then lower it. Repeat ten times on each side.

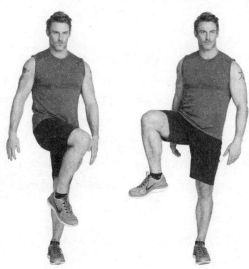

HALF JACKS

Set-up: Stand with arms by your sides.
Action: Tap your left leg out to your left side as you reach your right arm up to the ceiling. Repeat on the other side.

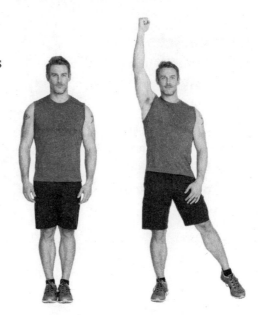

DAY 1: FITNESS ASSESSMENT (ALL LEVELS) AND SLOW-BURN CARDIO

Strength

You will need a stopwatch, a mat and a bench or sturdy chair. You will also need a pen and paper to record your repetitions and time held.

Perform each exercise for 30 seconds (except Plank, which you hold for as long as you can while timing yourself), count each repetition as you do it and then write it down. Now rest for 60 seconds before moving on to the next exercise.

Once you have recorded all exercises, total the number and divide by 4. Your total score determines whether you should do the beginner, intermediate or advanced workout:

Beginner: 0–29
Intermediate: 30–35
Advanced: 35+

For example, you do:

Press-ups: 15 reps

Plank: Held for 65 seconds

Squat: 12 reps

Triceps dips: 16 reps

Total: 108

Divide the total number by 4 to get 27. This person will perform the Beginner strength workouts.

Instructions for Strength exercises

PRESS-UPS

Set-up: Lie on the floor on your stomach, with your hands close to your chest and your elbows at a 45-degree angle.

Action: Raise yourself off the floor until your arms are fully extended. Your hands and the balls of your feet should support your weight. Keep a straight line from your head to your heels, contracting your abdominals and glutes so that your hips don't sag. Lower your chest to the floor. Repeat.

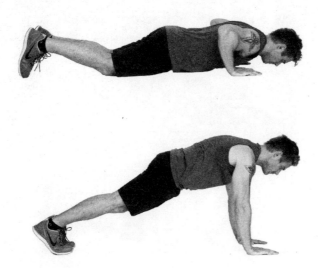

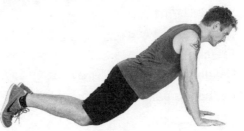

If you need to perform press-ups on your knees, subtract 5 from the total number of press-ups.

SQUATS (see page 106 for photos)

Set-up: Stand with your feet hip-width apart, arms at your sides.
Action: Bend your knees as though you're sitting down in a chair until your thighs are nearly parallel to the floor. Slowly return to start position.

PLANK

Set-up: Get into a press-up position, bend your elbows and bring your weight onto your forearms instead of your hands.
Action: Brace your abdominal muscles and keep a straight line from your shoulders to your ankles. Record how long you can hold plank with good form (see page 191). *If you need to perform the plank on your knees, subtract 15 from the total number of seconds held.*

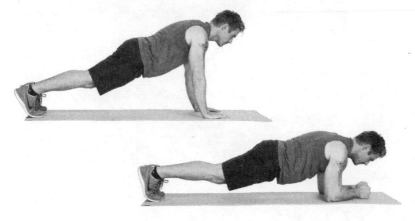

TRICEPS DIPS

Set-up: Sit on the edge of a bench or sturdy chair, hands grasping the seat on either side of your hips. Keep feet flat on the floor with your knees bent, and bring your hips off the edge of the bench or chair.

Action: Bend your elbows and lower your hips towards the floor. Straighten your arms and return to the start position.

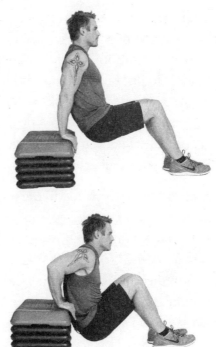

Day 1, part 2: Light cardio

You'll probably be moving more than you used to on The Programme. During the first four Cleanse days, while you're eating pretty lightly, you'll do about 20 minutes of light cardio exercise in addition to the daily fitness assessments. After the first four days of The Programme, you'll be doing a more intense Wake Up workout each morning and a workout routine associated with one of the assessed fitness areas every day, but you can also continue to walk or run on any or all of the remaining Programme days; many people find they really enjoy it. For today, it's just the assessment and the walk or run. There's no test: I'm relying on you to give yourself a reasonable challenge if you choose to take it. Do the warm up on page 144 and then spend 20 minutes in motion today in one of the following ways:

Beginner If you have been completely or primarily sedentary before beginning The Programme, set aside 20 minutes to walk. Don't worry about how far or fast you go during that time, the point is to just get back into motion and see how you feel. Our bodies were made to walk, and you don't require any training background to do it. Just put on a comfortable pair of shoes and get outside. Take some water with you if you think you'll need it. Enjoy your walk, and slow down or rest if you feel breathless.

Intermediate If you feel like just walking for 20 minutes would be no big deal for you, try walking that amount of time briskly. If you have a timer and/or step tracker on your phone or wrist-watch, try using it and see if you can cover a mile and a half in 20 minutes. Walking a mile in about 15 minutes is brisk. You shouldn't be feeling overwhelmed, but you'll get a bit more of a workout and start recruiting a higher percentage of your slow-twitch muscle fibres.

Advanced You can spend your 20 minutes alternating walking with jogging at a very comfortable pace. Start by walking for a few minutes, then jog at a pace where you could still have a conversation with someone. When you feel like you're working too hard to do that, or even if you're just noticing that you're breathing pretty heavily, slow down to a walk and keep walking until you feel completely recovered. Pick up the jog again when you feel ready. You might alternate between walking and jogging four times each in 20 minutes, or even ten times, whatever is comfortable for you.

If you are already pretty fit, jog continuously for 20 minutes each day during the Cleanse portion of The Programme. You are not sprinting, don't worry about your pace at all. You just want a comfortable, easy jog on relatively flat ground. If you feel breathless after 10 or 15 minutes, feel free to slow down to a brisk walk until you are completely recovered and then resume jogging.

Whatever you decide to do, if you feel spent, breathless and exhausted at the end of your 20 minutes, go down a level tomorrow. The point here is to be in motion, not push it to the max. The feeling you're going for is to be energised and refreshed after some mild activity, and perhaps to be excited to do it again tomorrow. You should ideally feel like you could have kept going for another 10 minutes, because after four days of this you'll be primed for more intense exercise.

DAY 2: FITNESS ASSESSMENT (ALL LEVELS)

Athletic

You will need a stopwatch, a clear area to move in (ideally not carpeted) and a pen and paper to record your repetitions.

Perform each exercise for 30 seconds, count each repetition as you do it, and then write the number down. Rest for 60 seconds before moving on to the next exercise. Once you have recorded your scores for all exercises, total the number and divide it by 4. Your total score determines whether you should do the beginner, intermediate or advanced workout:

Beginner: 0–24
Intermediate: 25–34
Advanced: 35+

For example, if you do:
Side shuffles: 25
Skipping: 35
Pass the ball, shoot the ball: 17
Speed skate: 27
Total: 104
Divide the total number by 4 to get 26. This person will do the Intermediate athletic workouts.

Instructions for Athletic exercises

SIDE SHUFFLES

Set-up: Stand with your feet shoulder-width apart, knees slightly bent.

Action: Take a large step out to your left with your left foot, bring your right foot out to meet the left. Take another large step to the left with your left foot then bend your knees and tap the floor with your right hand. Repeat in the other direction. One repetition is counted for each tap.

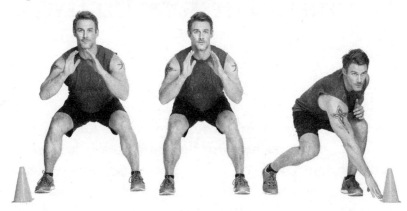

SKIPPING RIGHT/LEFT

Set-up: Stand with your feet together and imagine you are holding skipping-rope handles.

Action: Push off the floor with the balls of your feet and jump softly to your right. Push off again and jump softly to your left.

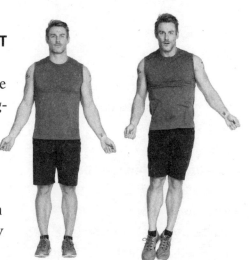

PASS THE BALL, SHOOT THE BALL

Set-up: Stand with your feet slightly wider than hip-width apart, knees slightly bent and hands at chest level.

Action: Imagine you are holding a football at your chest; pivot to your left side and push your arms out as if passing the ball. Come back to starting position and jump up or lift up on your toes and pretend to shoot the ball. Repeat on the other side. One rep is counted for each time you shoot the ball. *If you are lifting on your toes instead of jumping, subtract 10 from the total number of repetitions.*

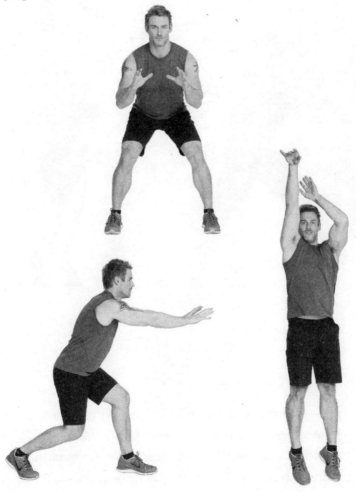

SPEED SKATE

Set-up: Stand with your feet hip-width apart, knees slightly bent.
Action: Leap or step to the left side and land on your left leg, reach across with your right hand towards your left knee or toes. Leap or step to the right side and land on your right leg, reaching across with your left hand.

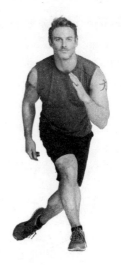

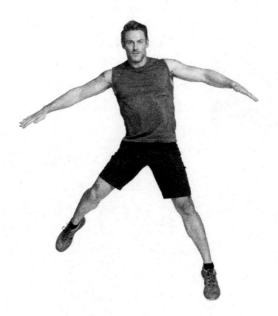

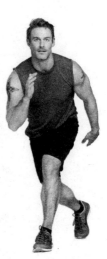

Part 2: Light cardio

Walk or jog for 20 minutes, following the instructions from Day 1. If you were very tired after what you did yesterday, go down a level. If you feel like you could have gone harder, feel free to try the next level up. Remember, the point is simply to enjoy being in motion today, not to push it really hard. If you are sore, go down a level (or walk for a shorter distance if you are a beginner) but don't skip this exercise: the kind of walking I'm asking you to do is good for sore muscles and will make you feel better than simply resting.

DAY 3: FITNESS ASSESSMENT (ALL LEVELS)

Metabolic

You will need a stopwatch, and a sturdy wall to lean against. You will also need a pen and paper to record your repetitions/ time held.

Perform each exercise for 30 seconds (except for the wall sit, which is held for as long as possible), count each repetition as you do it, and then write it down and rest for 60 seconds before moving on to the next exercise.

Once you have recorded all exercises, total the number and divide by 4. Your score determines whether you should do the beginner, intermediate or advanced workout.

Beginner: 0–30
Intermediate: 30–50
Advanced: 50+

For example, if you do:
Squat thrusts: 15
High knee jog: 43
Wall sit: 110 seconds
Alternating lateral lunges: 18
Total: 186
Divide the total number by 4 to get 46. This person will do the Intermediate metabolic workout

Instructions for metabolic exercises

SQUAT THRUSTS

Set-up: Stand with your feet together, arms at your sides.

Action: Bend your knees and place your palms on the floor with your arms on the outside of your knees. Shift your weight onto your palms. Jump both feet back and land in plank position or walk one foot at a time into plank position. Jump both feet forwards and return to standing. *If you need to step into plank, subtract 5 from the total number of repetitions.*

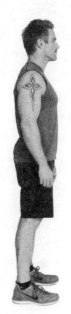

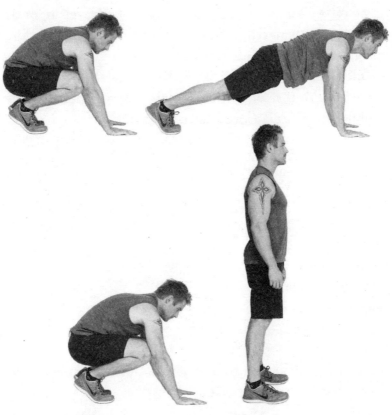

HIGH KNEE JOG

Set-up: Stand with your feet hip-width apart, knees slightly bent, and elbows bent 90 degrees. *Action:* Bring your left knee up to hip level, push off your right foot and change legs, bringing your right leg up to hip level. Continue running in place and touching your hand to your thighs each time your leg comes up.

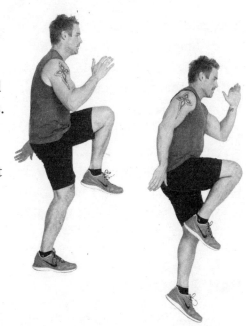

ALTERNATING LATERAL LUNGES

Set-up: Stand with your feet together, hands on your hips.
Action: Take a big step to the left, keeping your right toes pointing straight ahead, and bend your left knee until your thigh is almost parallel to the floor. Keep your right knee straight, but not locked. Press off your left foot to return to start position. Repeat on the other leg.

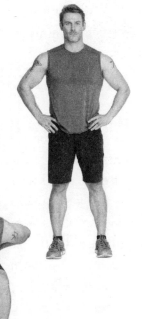

WALL SIT

Set-up: Stand with your back against a wall, placing your feet about 60cm (2ft) in front of you. Your feet should be hip-width apart.

Action: Bend your knees and slide down the wall until your knees are at 90-degree angles. Your knees should be over your ankles, and your thighs parallel to the floor. Place your palms on the wall.

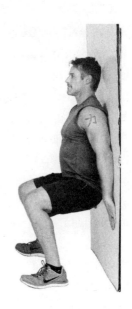

Part 2: Light cardio

Walk or jog for 20 minutes, following the instructions from Day 1. Feel free to mix it up by going down or up a level depending on how you feel, and remember that the point is to just enjoy being in motion today.

DAY 4: FITNESS ASSESSMENT (ALL LEVELS)

Part 1: Slow Burn

This slow-burn exercise assesses your current aerobic endurance. You will need an outdoor area where you can walk, jog or run, or a treadmill. This is a little different from the way I have asked you to walk or jog over the last three days (you'll still need to do that as well), because I want you to record the distance you cover in 10 minutes. If you want to continue walking or jogging for an additional 10 minutes and call that your cardio for the day, you can, or you can take this test and then go for a 20-minute walk or jog without worrying about recording anything later in the day, it's up to you.

Set-up: Begin with a 3-minute walk at a comfortable pace.
Action: Walk, jog or run for 10 minutes. Record the distance. For example, you might record two laps around a standard track or half a mile in 10 minutes. There are many apps you can download on your phone to do this if you don't have a good sense of the distance on your own.

The distance you cover determines your level of fitness at steady-state cardio activities. If you can do two laps around a standard track or half a mile in 10 minutes, you should do the intermediate level of the Slow Burn and Flow workout. If that isn't achievable, do the beginner level Slow Burn and Flow workout; if it's relatively easy, go for the advanced level workout.

Part 2: Flow

The Flow is a series of five yoga postures to increase your range of motion: Downward-facing Dog, Low Lunge, Warrior I, Warrior II and Side Angle. These poses focus on stretching the major muscle groups you will be using during your workouts (chest, shoulders, thighs, hip flexors and back). You are not scoring yourself on these poses – you just want to learn how to do them on day 4, see how they feel, then use this series as a cool-down after your regular workouts, or at any point that you want to work on increasing your flexibility. *You will need a yoga mat.*

Instructions for Flow exercises

DOWNWARD-FACING DOG
Set-up: Begin in plank position. As you inhale, spread your fingers wide and press both palms firmly into the mat while

simultaneously tucking your toes under. As you exhale, begin to draw your hips towards the ceiling, making the shape of an inverted V. Your head and neck should be between your upper arms. Bend your knees as much as you need to while maintaining equal weight on your hands and feet. Hold for three to five breath cycles.

Flow from Downward-facing Dog into Low Lunge.

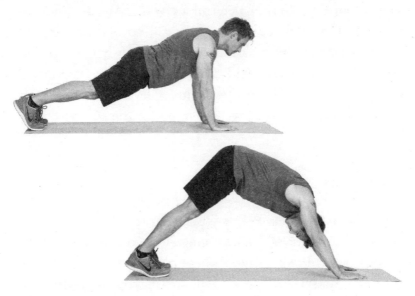

LOW LUNGE

Step your left foot between your hands, shifting your weight forwards slightly to allow your left thigh to become parallel to the floor while remaining on the ball of your back foot (your right foot).

Flow from Low Lunge into Warrior I.

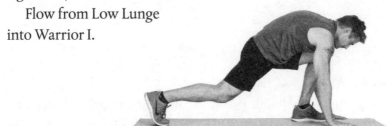

WARRIOR I

Keeping your front foot facing forwards, turn your back foot slightly outward and let your back foot rest flat at a 45-degree angle. Reach your arms over your head so that they are parallel to one another. Your hips should still be facing forwards. Lower your shoulder away from your ears and lift your core as you bend your front knee (your left knee) into a 90-degree angle.

Hold for three to five breath cycles.

Flow from Warrior I into Warrior II.

WARRIOR II

Rotate your weight to the left and bring your arms straight out to your sides, parallel to the floor. The position of your feet does not change, but your hips should be in line with your shoulders. Your front leg (your left leg) should be bent while your back (right) leg is straight. Hold for three to five breath cycles.

Flow from Warrior II into Side Angle.

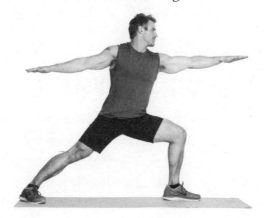

SIDE ANGLE

Drop your left forearm on to your left thigh and tilt your torso open, so that your right hand is now up in the air, reaching for the ceiling. Hold for three to five breath cycles.

Repeat this sequence on the other side. This means that from Downward Dog you'll step your right leg forward and repeat the entire flow on your right side.

Continue to alternate sides, two to five times.

Part 3: Light cardio

If you did not extend the Slow-burn assessment to walk or jog for an additional 10 minutes, make sure you also do a 20-minute walk or jog today, following the instructions from Day 1. Feel free to mix it up by going down or up a level depending on how you feel and remember that the point of this one is simply to enjoy being in motion. You'll start the workouts tomorrow, so don't overdo it!

BONUS WORKOUT: 5 CORE STRENGTH EXERCISES

Many of my clients want to focus on their core strength or to target weight loss in that area. There are many ways of moving that strengthen the core, and everything you're doing in the workouts during The Programme will help you lose weight. But if you're interested in doing some extra moves, consider adding these to your routine or fitting in this little workout in the same way that you might make time for a quick stretch workout if you're working on flexibility.

Beginner Perform 10 reps of each exercise, rest for 30 seconds, then move on to the next exercise. Repeat the circuit three times.

Intermediate Perform 20 reps of each exercise, rest for 30 seconds, then move on to the next exercise. Repeat the circuit three times.

Advanced Perform 30 reps of each exercise, rest for 30 seconds, then move on to the next exercise. Repeat the circuit three times.

Between each set perform eight stability ball back extensions (instructions page 167).

1. CRUNCH

Set-up: Lie face-up with your knees bent, feet flat on the floor, and hands behind your head with fingertips by your ears.
Action: Lift your shoulders off the floor until you feel a tight contraction on your abdominals. Return to starting position and repeat.

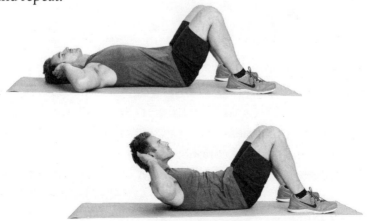

2. REVERSE CRUNCHES

Set-up: Lie face-up on the floor. Place both hands by your hips, palms down.

Action: Keeping your knees and ankles together, bring your knees towards your chest. Squeeze your abdominals to lift your hips and legs towards the ceiling. Lower your legs and repeat.

JESSIE'S TIP *Don't use your legs as momentum to lift up. Focus on the power coming from your abs.*

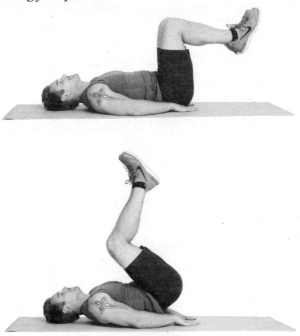

3. STABILITY BALL CRUNCH (see opposite above)

Set-up: Sit on the ball, walk forward and rest your lower back on the ball. Bend your knees and keep your feet flat on the floor. Place your hands behind your head.

Action: Contract your abdominals to lift your torso off the ball, drawing your belly button towards your spine. Return to the start position.

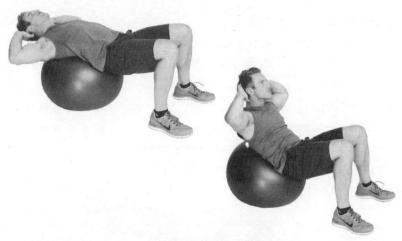

4. STABILITY BALL OBLIQUE CRUNCH

Set-up: Sit on the ball, walk forward and rest your lower back on the ball. Bend your knees and keep your feet flat on the floor. Place your left hand behind your head and your right hand at your navel. *Action:* Contract your abdominals to lift your torso off the ball, and twist over towards your right knee, drawing your belly button towards your spine. Return to start position. Repeat all reps, then change sides.

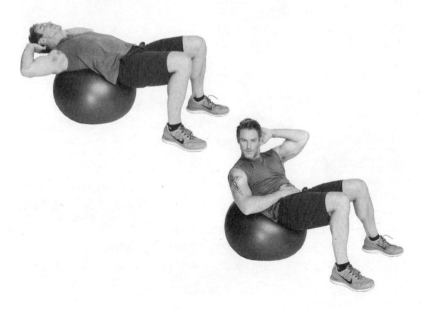

5. STABILITY BALL PIKE

Set-up: Start with your torso on the ball and hands and feet on the floor. Walk your hands forward until your ankles are on top of the ball.

Action: Keeping your legs straight, pull your feet towards your chest, raise your hips towards the ceiling as the ball rolls in, and continue until your hips are directly under your shoulders. Slowly lower back to starting position.

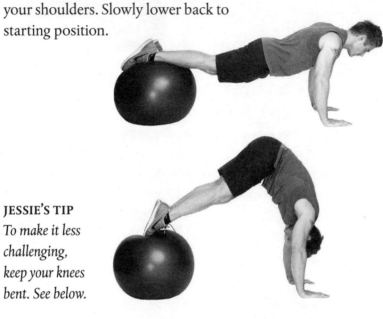

JESSIE'S TIP
To make it less challenging, keep your knees bent. See below.

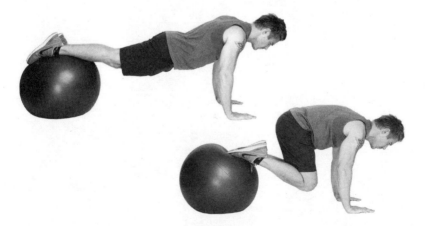

Between each set perform eight back extensions (instructions below).

STABILITY BALL BACK EXTENSION

Set-up: Lie face-down on a stability ball with your hands on the ball at your sides, about 15cm (6 inches) apart. Press your feet against a wall or sturdy object.

Action: Lift your torso up until your body forms a straight line.

JESSIE'S TIP *To make it more challenging, perform the exercise with your fingertips by your ears instead of on the ball.*

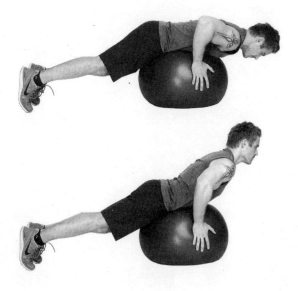

BEGINNER WORKOUTS

Beginner Wake-Up workout

Starting on Day 5, do the following 4-minute circuit every day, to get you ready and energised for a healthy day. Do each exercise for 20 seconds, recover for 10 seconds and then move on to the next exercise. Repeat the circuit two times.

Beginner
Jumping Jacks or Half Jacks
Squats
Knee Press-ups
Reverse Lunges

JUMPING JACKS
Set-up: Stand with your arms by your sides.
Action: Jump your legs out to the sides as you bring your arms overhead. Jump your feet back together and return your arms to your sides.

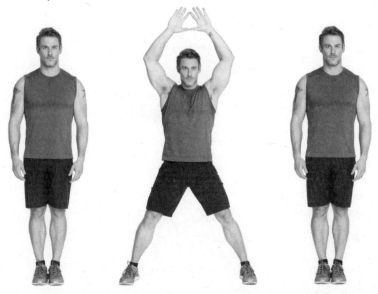

HALF JACKS

Set-up: Start standing with your arms by your sides.
Action: Tap your left leg out to the left side as you lift your right arm up to the ceiling. Repeat on the other side.

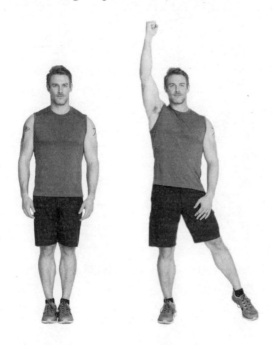

SQUATS (see page 106 for photos)

Set-up: Stand with your feet hip-width apart, arms by your sides.
Action: Bend your knees as though you're sitting down in a chair until your thighs are nearly parallel to the floor. Slowly return to start position

KNEE PRESS-UPS (see page 148 for photos)

Set-up: Start on your hands and knees. Straighten your torso, place your hands underneath your shoulders, but slightly wider than your shoulders, and rest on your knees.
Action: Bend your elbows and slowly lower your chest towards the floor. Push up to start position.

REVERSE LUNGES

Set-up: Stand with your feet shoulder-width apart.

Action: Take a step backwards with your right leg, lowering the right knee towards the floor. Push off the right foot to come back to start position. Repeat alternating legs.

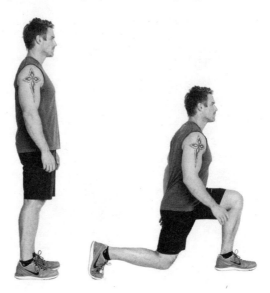

Day 5 BURN: Metabolic training

5 exercises   1 minute each   6 sets

Perform each exercise for 60 seconds and then move on to the next exercise. Complete one set, recover for 90 seconds, then repeat, making six sets in total.

SQUAT WITH DUMB-BELL OVERHEAD PRESS

Set-up: Stand with your feet hip-width apart, holding a dumb-bell in each hand at your shoulders, palms facing in.

Action: Bend your knees as though you're sitting down in a chair until your thighs are nearly parallel to the floor. As you rise out of the squat, lift the dumb-bells overhead until they are about 2cm (1 inch) apart. Lower the dumb-bells as you return to start position.

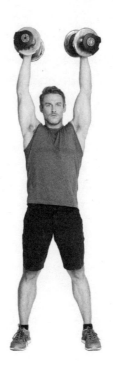

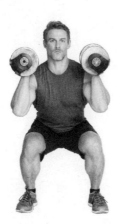

ALTERNATING STEP-UPS

Set-up: Stand with your feet hip-width apart in front of a bench.

Action: Place your right foot firmly on the bench. Push through your right heel to raise your body onto the bench, tap your left foot to the top of the bench, return to start position and step up with your left foot. Continue alternating legs.

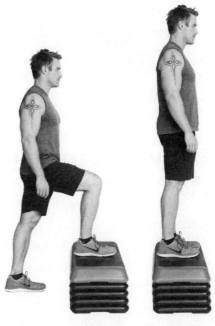

SUMO SQUAT BICEPS CURL

Set-up: Stand with feet slightly wider than hip-width apart, toes out, holding a dumb-bell in each hand, palms facing in.

Action: Bend your knees and lower your body until your thighs are parallel to the floor. Push yourself back up as you rotate your wrists outwards and curl the dumb-bells to your shoulders.

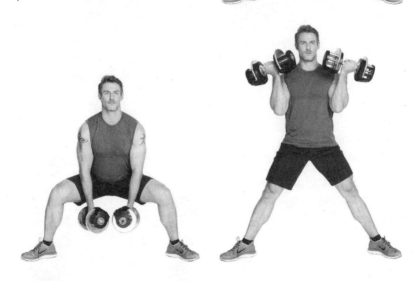

REVERSE LUNGE LATERAL RAISE (see opposite above)

Set-up: Stand with your feet shoulder-width apart, holding a dumb-bell in each hand, arms by your sides, palms facing each other.

Action: Take a step backwards with your right leg, lowering your right knee towards the floor, simultaneously lifting dumb-bells out to the sides to shoulder level. Return to start position and continue alternating legs.

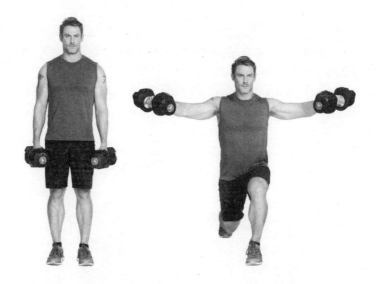

CRUNCH (see page 163 for photos)

Set-up: Lie face up with your knees bent, feet flat on the floor and your hands behind your head, with fingertips lightly touching.

Action: Lift your shoulders off the floor until you feel a tight contraction in your abdominals. Return to start position and repeat.

Day 6 BUILD: Strength training

Push day

7 exercises   5 reps   5 sets

Perform each exercise five times and then move on to the next exercise. Recover for 30–60 seconds between sets.

KNEE PRESS-UPS (see page 148 for photos)

Set-up: Start on your hands and knees. Straighten your torso, place your hands underneath your shoulders, but slightly wider than your shoulders, and rest on your knees.

Action: Bend your elbows and slowly lower your chest towards the floor. Push up to start position.

SHOULDER PRESS

Set-up: Stand with feet shoulder-width apart, holding a dumb-bell in each hand at shoulder level.

Action: Press dumb-bells overhead, keeping your arms in line with your ears. Slowly lower your arms to shoulder height.

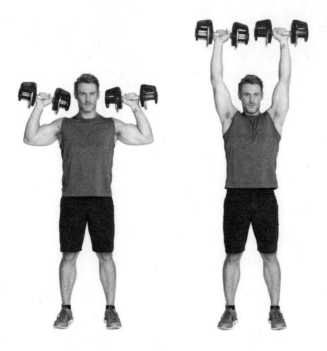

TRICEPS DIPS (see page 149 for photos)

Set-up: Sit on the edge of a bench or sturdy chair, hands grasping the seat on either side of your hips. Keep your feet flat on the floor with your knees bent and bring your hips off the edge of the bench or chair.

Action: Bend your elbows and lower your hips towards the floor. Straighten your arms and return to starting position.

LATERAL RAISES

Set-up: Stand with your feet shoulder-width apart, holding a dumb-bell in each hand, palms facing in.

Action: Keeping arms straight, but not locked, raise the dumb-bells out to the side in line with your shoulders. Lower the dumb-bells to starting position.

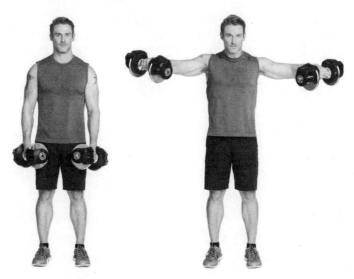

DUMB-BELL CHEST FLY

Set-up: Lie on an exercise bench or mat with a dumb-bell in each hand, palms facing in. Extend the dumb-bells over your chest.
Action: Lower your arms until the weights are even with your chest. Press the dumb-bells back to starting position.

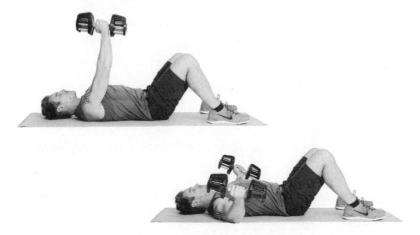

Day 7 BURN: Athletic training

HIIT (high intensity interval training)

4 exercises   30 seconds each   5 sets

Perform each exercise for 30 seconds, recover for 30 seconds, then move on to the next exercise.

Recover for 1 minute. Do the sets five times in total.

PASS THE BALL, SHOOT THE BALL (see page 153 for photos)
Set-up: Stand with your feet slightly wider than hip-width apart, knees slightly bent and hands at chest level.
Action: Imagine you are holding a football at your chest; pivot to your right side and push your arms out as if passing the ball. Come back to starting position and lift up on your toes or jump up and pretend to shoot the ball. Repeat on the other side.

SIDE SHUFFLES (see page 152 for photos)
Set-up: Stand with your feet shoulder-width apart, knees slightly bent.
Action: Take a large step out to your right with your right foot, bring your left foot out to meet the right. Take another large step to the left with your left foot then bend your knees and tap the floor with your right hand. Repeat in the other direction.

LUNGE KICK LUNGE (see opposite above)
Set-up: Stand with feet shoulder-width apart, knees slightly bent.
Action: Step back with your right foot into a lunge, press off the ball of your right foot and kick your right leg forward. Repeat for 30 seconds; switch sides on the next circuit.

JESSIE'S TIP *Don't worry about how high you kick, focus on your balance and keeping your core engaged.*

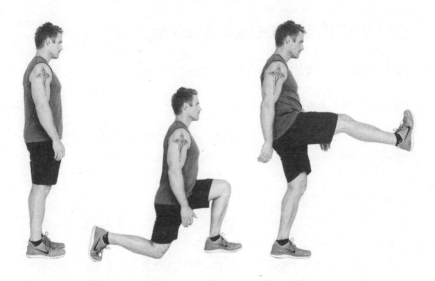

ALTERNATING ELBOW TO KNEE

Set-up: Stand with your feet shoulder-width apart, hands by your head.

Action: Lower your left elbow and raise your right knee, crunching them together on a diagonal line. Repeat for 30 seconds; switch sides on the next circuit.

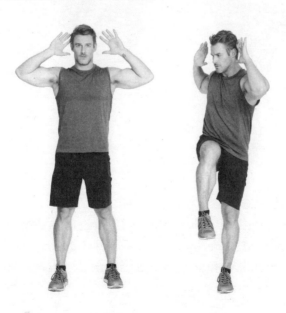

Day 8 BUILD: Strength training

Pull day

5 exercises   5 reps   5 sets

Perform each exercise five times and then move on to the next exercise. Recover for 30–60 seconds between sets.

DUMB-BELL ROW

Set-up: Stand with your feet hip-width apart, holding a dumb-bell in each hand, palms facing each other. Hinge forward to a 45-degree angle from the hips, keeping your back long and knees slightly bent.

Action: Pull the dumb-bells up until your elbows pass your torso; lower to starting position.

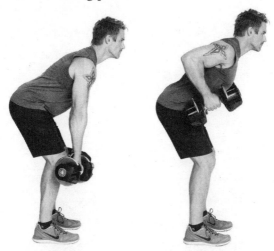

BICEPS CURLS (see opposite above)

Set-up: Stand with your feet hip-width apart, holding a dumb-bell in each hand, arms by your sides, palms facing in.

Action: Curl the weights towards your shoulders; lower to starting position.

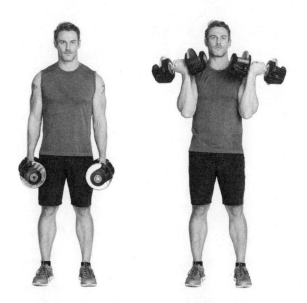

LAT PULLOVER

Set-up: Lie face-up on a bench or mat, holding a dumb-bell in each hand over your chest, keeping your elbows slightly bent.

Action: Extend your arms over your chest, palms facing in. Keeping your elbows slightly bent, lower the weights in an arc back over your head towards the floor. Bring your elbows level with your head and return to the start position.

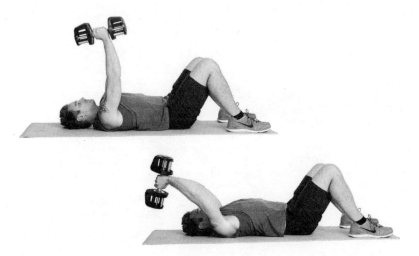

RESISTANCE BAND ROWS

Set-up: Attach the resistance band door attachment to chest height. Stand facing the door, holding both handles, with knees slightly bent.

Action: Reach forward with your arms in line with your shoulders. Pull the band back until your elbows pass your torso. Return to start.

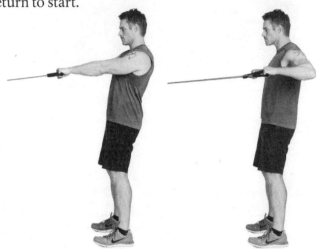

BACK EXTENSION WITH ALTERNATING ARM RAISE

Set-up: Lie face down on a mat with your arms and legs extended.

Action: Keeping your neck in line with your spine, lift your right leg and left arm off the mat. Return to start position and repeat on the other side.

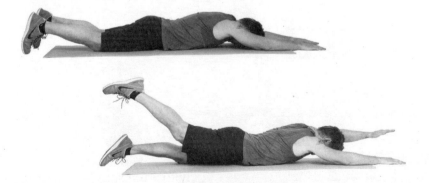

Day 9 BURN: Metabolic training

5 exercises   1 minute each   4 sets

Perform each exercise for 60 seconds, and then move on to the next exercise. Complete one set, recover for 90 seconds, then repeat, making four sets in total.

ALTERNATING LATERAL RAISE WITH LEG RAISE

Set-up: Stand with your feet shoulder-width apart, holding a dumb-bell in your left hand, both palms facing in.

Action: Raise your right leg out to the side, as you lift your left arm to the side until dumb-bell is shoulder level. Lower the dumb-bell as you return to start position. Repeat for 30 seconds and then switch sides.

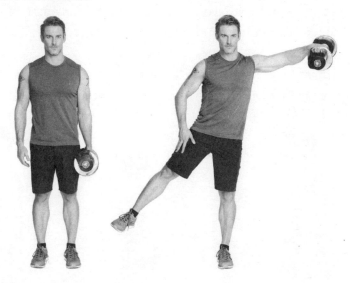

DUMB-BELL CHEST FLY WITH GLUTE BRIDGE

Set-up: Lie on an exercise bench or mat with your knees bent. Hold a dumb-bell in each hand, palms facing in. Extend the dumb-bells over your chest.

Action: Raise your hips so that body forms a straight line from your shoulder to your knees. Lower your hips back to the mat as you lower the dumb-bells until they are even with your chest.

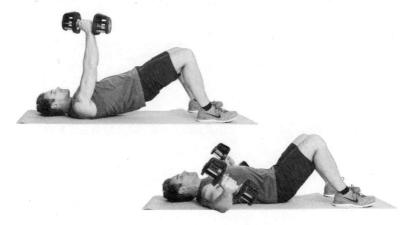

REVERSE LUNGE WITH OVERHEAD PRESS

Set-up: Stand with your feet shoulderwidth apart, holding a dumb-bell in each hand, arms by your sides, palms facing each other.

Action: Curl the dumb-bells up to your shoulders as you step your right foot back into a lunge. Press the dumb-bells overhead,

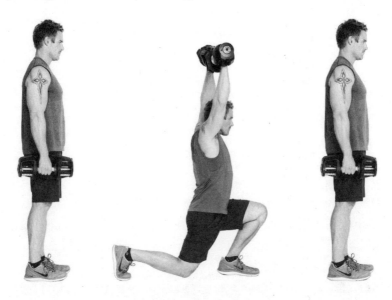

then press into your left heel to return to standing. Repeat for 30 seconds and then switch sides.

QUADRUPED HIP EXTENSION

Set-up: Start on your hands and knees, with your hands under your shoulders and your knees under your hips.

Action: Lift right leg behind you, keeping knee bent at a 90-degree angle and pressing your right foot towards the ceiling. Lower to start position. Repeat for 30 seconds and then switch sides.

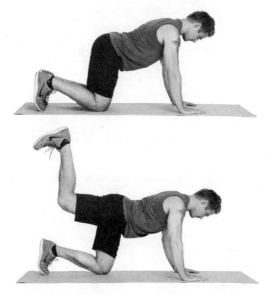

REVERSE CRUNCHES (see page 164 for photos)

Set-up: Lie face-up on the floor. Place both hands by your hips, palms down.

Action: Keeping your knees and ankles together, bring both knees towards your chest. Squeeze your abdominals to lift your hips and legs towards the ceiling.

Lower your legs and repeat.

JESSIE'S TIP *Don't use your legs as momentum to lift up, focus on the power coming from your abs.*

Day 10 BUILD: Strength training

Leg day

5 exercises   5 reps   5 sets

Perform each exercise five times and then move on to the next exercise. Recover for 30–60 seconds between sets.

SQUATS (see page 106 for photos)
Set-up: Stand with your feet hip-width apart, arms by your sides.
Action: Bend your knees as though you're sitting down in a chair until your thighs are nearly parallel to the floor. Slowly return to start position.

ALTERNATING LATERAL LUNGES
Set-up: Stand with your feet together, hands on hips.
Action: Take a big step to the left, keeping your right toes pointing straight ahead, and bending your left knee until your thigh is almost parallel to the floor. Keep your right knee straight, but

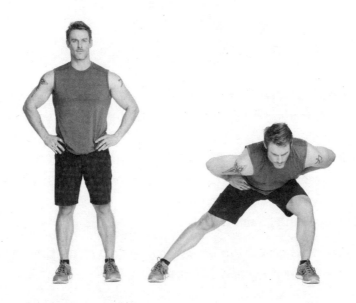

not locked. Press off your left foot to return to start position. Complete all reps then switch sides.

DEAD LIFT (see page 107 for photos)
Set-up: Stand with your feet shoulder-width apart, toes pointing straight ahead, arms by your sides, and palms facing your thighs.
Action: Keeping your back straight, hinge forward at your hips and lower your torso until it's almost parallel to the floor. Contract your hamstrings and glutes and push your hips forward to return to standing.

QUADRUPED HIP EXTENSION (see page 183 for photos)
Set-up: Start on your hands and knees, with your hands under your shoulders and your knees under your hips.
Action: Lift right leg behind you, keeping knee bent at a 90-degree angle and pressing your right foot towards the ceiling. Return to start. Repeat for 30 seconds, then switch sides.

GLUTE BRIDGE
Set-up: Lie on your back with your knees bent and your feet flat on the floor.
Action: Lift your hips off the floor, press your heels into the floor and contract your glutes. Lower to start position.

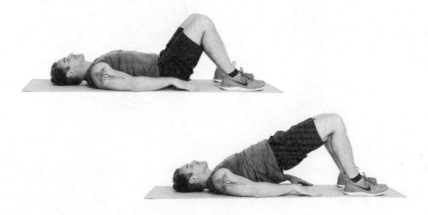

Day 11 BURN: Athletic training

HIIT athletic training

5 exercises   30 seconds each   5 sets

Do each exercise for 30 seconds, recover for 30 seconds, then move on to the next exercise.

Recover for 1 minute, then repeat, making five sets in total.

REVERSE LUNGE WITH ROTATION
Set-up: Stand with your feet shoulder-width apart, with finger-tips by your ears.
Action: Take a step backwards with your left leg, lowering your left knee towards the floor; keeping your hips facing forwards and chest open, twist to the right. Return to face forwards and then push back to starting position. Continue alternating legs.

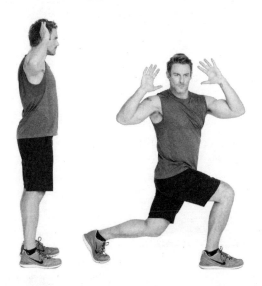

SKIPPING (see page 152 for photos)
Set-up: Stand with feet together; imagine you are holding skipping rope handles.

Action: Push off the floor with the balls of your feet, land softly and push off again.

SPEED SKATE (see page 154 for photos)
Set-up: Stand with your feet hip-width apart, knees slightly bent.
Action: Leap or step to the left side and land on your left leg, reach across with your right hand towards your left knee or toes. Repeat on the other side.

JUMPING JACKS (see page 168 for photos)
Set-up: Stand with your arms by your sides.
Action: Jump your legs out to the sides as you bring your arms overhead.
Jump your feet back together and return arms to your sides.

HALF JACKS are an easier version (see page 169 for photos)
Set-up: Start standing with your arms by your sides. Tap your left leg out to your right side as you reach your right arm up to the ceiling.
Action: Repeat on the other side.

Day 12 BUILD: Strength training

Full body

5 exercises   5 reps   5 sets

Perform each exercise five times and then move on to the next exercise. Recover for 30–60 seconds between sets.

SQUAT WITH KNEE RAISE BALANCE
Set-up: Stand with your feet hip-width apart, arms by your sides.
Action: Bend your knees as though you're sitting down in a chair

until your thighs are nearly parallel to the floor; keeping your weight on your left foot, raise your right knee towards your chest as you stand up. Return to squat position. Repeat 5 times on right side and then 5 times on the left side.

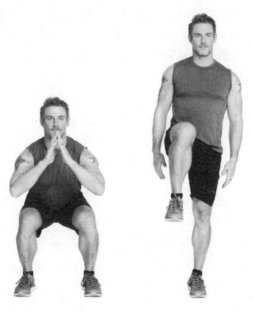

KNEE PRESS-UPS (see page 148 for photos)
Set-up: Start on your hands and knees. Straighten your torso, place your hands underneath your shoulders, but slightly wider than your shoulders, and rest on your knees.
Action: Bend your elbows and slowly lower your chest towards the floor. Push up to start position.

REVERSE LUNGE WITH ROTATION (see page 186 for photos)
Set-up: Stand with your feet shoulder-width apart, with finger-tips by your ears.
Action: Take a step backwards with your left leg, lowering left knee towards the floor; keeping your hips facing forwards and chest open, twist to the right. Return to face forwards and then

push back to starting position. Repeat 5 times on left side and then 5 times on the right side.

DUMB-BELL CHEST FLY WITH GLUTE BRIDGE
(see page 181 for photos)

Set-up: Lie on an exercise bench or mat with your knees bent and your feet flat on the floor. Hold a dumb-bell in each hand, palms facing in. Extend the dumb-bells over your chest.

Action: Raise your hips so your body forms a straight line from your shoulders to your knees. Lower your hips back to the mat as you lower the dumb-bells until they are even with your chest.

SQUAT WITH DUMB-BELL OVERHEAD PRESS
(see page 195 for photos)

Set-up: Stand with your feet hip-width apart, holding a dumb-bell in each hand at your shoulders, palms facing in.

Action: Bend your knees as though you're sitting down in a chair until your thighs are nearly parallel to the floor. As you rise out of the squat, lift the dumb-bells overhead until they are about 2cm (1 inch) apart. Lower the dumb-bells as you return to start position.

Day 13: Slow Burn and Flow

Slow Burn

Walk briskly or jog for 20 minutes today. This should be at a somewhat higher intensity than you were able to do during the first four Cleanse eating days. If you have a timer or step tracker on your phone or wristwatch, try using it and see if you can cover 1½ miles in 20 minutes. One mile in about 15 minutes is very brisk. If you are able to, intersperse your brisk walking with a light jog when you can. Start by walking for a few minutes, then jog at a pace such that you could still have a conversation with someone. When you feel like you're working too hard to do that, or even if you're noticing that you're breathing heavily, slow down to a walk and keep walking until you feel completely recovered. You might alternate between walking and jogging four times each in 20 minutes, or even 10 times – anything is fine.

Flow

The Flow exercise routine for Day 13 is the same sequence that you first performed on Day 4, so simply repeat that – see page 159 for instructions and photos.

DAYS 14 TO 21

During these days you repeat the sequences carried out on earlier days, as follows:

Day 14: repeat Day 6   (see page 196)

Day 15: repeat Day 7   (see page 199)

Day 16: repeat Day 8   (see page 201)

Day 17: repeat Day 5   (see page 170)

Day 18: repeat Day 10   (see page 184)

Day 19: repeat Day 11   (see page 186)

Day 20: repeat Day 12   (see page 187)

Day 21: repeat Day 9   (see page 181)

INTERMEDIATE WORKOUTS

Wake-Up workout

Starting on Day 5, do the following 4-minute circuit every day, to get you ready and energised for a healthy day. Do each exercise for 20 seconds, recover for 10 seconds and then move on to the next exercise. Repeat the circuit twice.

Intermediate
Jumping Jacks
Press-ups
Alternating Lateral Lunge
Plank with alternating knee cross

JUMPING JACKS (see page 168 for photos)
Set-up: Stand with your arms by your sides.
Action: Jump your legs out to the sides as you bring your arms overhead. Jump your feet back together and return arms to your sides.

PRESS-UPS (see page 147 for photos)
Set-up: Lie on the floor on your stomach, with your hands close to your chest and your elbows at a 45-degree angle.
Action: Raise yourself off the floor until your arms are fully extended. Your hands and the balls of your feet should support your weight. Keep a straight line from your head to your heels, contracting your abdominals and glutes so that your hips don't sag. Lower your chest to the floor and repeat.

ALTERNATING LATERAL LUNGES (see page 157 for photos)
Set-up: Stand with your feet shoulder-width apart, hands on hips.
Action: Take a big step to the left, keeping your right toes

pointing straight ahead, and bending your left knee until your thigh is almost parallel to the floor. Keep your right knee straight, but not locked. Press off your left foot to return to start position. Repeat on the other leg.

PLANK WITH KNEE CROSS

Set-up: Start in press-up position with hands directly under your shoulders.

Action: Turn your right knee in and bring it towards your left shoulder. Return to start position and repeat on the other side.

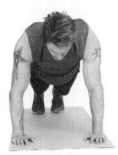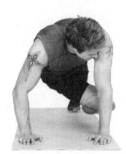

Day 5: BURN – Metabolic training

5 exercises   1 minute each   4 sets

Perform each exercise for 60 seconds then move on to the next exercise. Complete one circuit, recover for 90 seconds. Do the sets four times in total.

DUMB-BELL STEP-UP WITH BICEPS CURL

Set-up: Stand with your feet hip-width apart in front of a bench. Hold a dumb-bell in each hand, arms by your sides, palms facing in.

Action: Place your right foot firmly on the bench. Push through your right heel to raise your body onto the bench; as you lift up, curl the dumb-bells up towards your shoulders, with palms facing in; tap your left foot to the top of the bench; return to start position as you lower the dumb-bells. Repeat on the right side for 30 seconds then change sides.

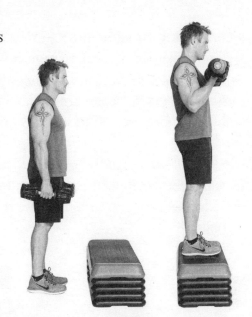

DUMB-BELL WOOD CHOP

Set-up: Stand with feet wider than hip-width apart, holding a dumb-bell with both hands high above your right shoulder, arms straight with a slight bend at your elbows. Rotate your torso to the right.

Action: Swing the dumb-bell down to the outside of your left knee as you rotate to the left, pivoting on your right toes and bending both knees. Return to start position and repeat for 30 seconds then change sides.

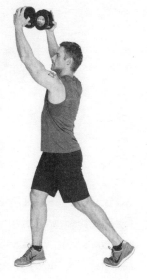

RESISTANCE BAND CHEST FLY

Set-up: Attach the resistance band door attachment at chest height. Stand with your back facing the door, one handle in each hand. Extend your arms out with your palms facing each other, step the right foot forward into a lunge until the band is taut.

Action: Pull your hands together, maintaining a slight bend in your elbows. Return to start and repeat for 30 seconds with the right leg forward, then switch legs and repeat for 30 seconds.

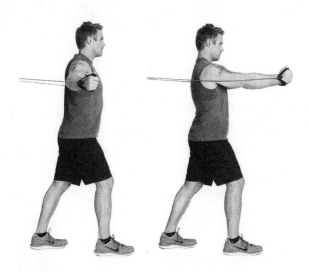

SQUAT WITH DUMB-BELL OVERHEAD PRESS

(See opposite above)

Set-up: Stand with your feet hip-width apart, holding a dumb-bell in each hand at your shoulders, palms facing in.

Action: Bend your knees as though you're sitting down in a chair until your thighs are nearly parallel to the floor. As you rise out of the squat, lift the dumb-bells overhead until they are about 2cm (1 inch) apart. Lower the dumb-bells as you return to start position.

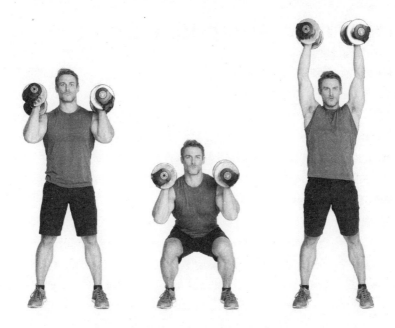

RUSSIAN TWIST WITH DUMB-BELL

Set-up: Sit on the floor with your knees bent and your heels about 30cm (12 inches) from your hips. Hold a dumb-bell with both hands in front of your chest. Lean back to a 45-degree angle without rounding your back.

Action: Holding the dumb-bell at your chest, with elbows bent, pull your navel in to your spine and rotate your torso to the right. Come back to centre and rotate left.

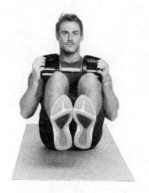
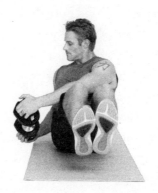

Day 6 BUILD: strength training

Push day

5 exercises   10 reps   4 sets

Perform each exercise ten times, and then move on to the next exercise. Recover for 30–60 seconds between sets.

PRESS-UPS (see page 147 for photos)
Set-up: Lie on the floor on your stomach, with your hands close to your chest and your elbows at a 45-degree angle.
Action: Raise yourself off the floor until your arms are fully extended; your hands and the balls of your feet should support your weight. Keep a straight line from your head to your heels, contracting your abdominals and glutes so that your hips don't sag. Lower your chest to the floor and repeat.

TRICEPS EXTENSION
Set-up: Stand with your feet shoulder-width apart, holding a dumb-bell in each hand.
Action: Lift the dumb-bells overhead and lower your hands behind your head, keeping your elbows close to your ears. Push the dumb-bells towards the ceiling without locking your elbows.

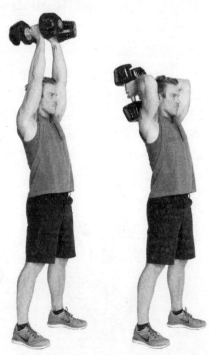

CHEST PRESS ON STABILITY BALL

Set-up: Sit on the stability ball holding a dumb-bell in each hand, with dumb-bells resting on your thighs. Slowly walk your feet forwards and slide your torso down the ball until your head, shoulders and upper back are on the ball. Feet are parallel and knees are shoulder-width apart, bent at 90 degrees so that your thighs and torso are parallel to the floor.

Action: Position the dumb-bells over your chest with your palms facing forwards. Press the dumb-bells upwards above your chest, elbows straight but not locked. Lower the dumb-bells until they are level with your chest. Return to starting position.

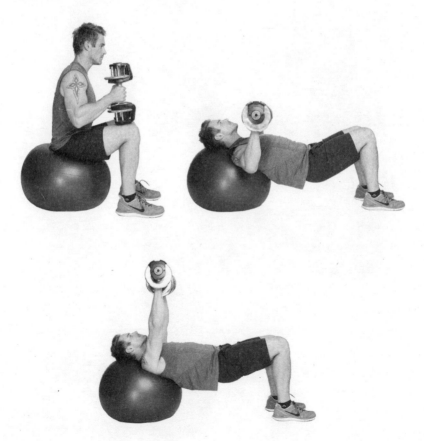

TRICEPS EXTENSION ON STABILITY BALL

Set-up: Sit on a stability ball with a dumb-bell in each hand, feet flat on the floor and dumb-bells resting on your thighs. Slowly walk your feet forwards and slide your torso down the ball until your head, shoulders and upper back are on the ball. Your feet are parallel and knees are shoulder-width apart, bent 90 degrees so that your thighs and torso are parallel to the floor.

Action: Extend your arms at a 90-degree angle from the floor. Bend your elbows so that your forearms are parallel to the floor. Straighten your arms without locking your elbows.

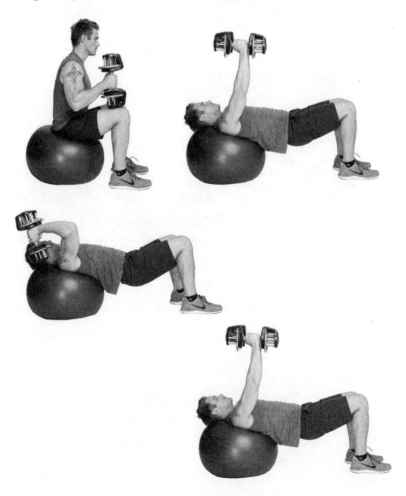

LATERAL RAISE (see page 222 for photos)

Set-up: Stand with your feet shoulder-width apart, holding a dumb-bell in each hand, palms facing each other.

Action: Keeping your elbows slightly bent, raise the dumb-bells to the sides until your arms are parallel to the floor; lower to start position.

Day 7 BURN: Athletic training

HIIT (high intensity interval training)

5 exercises   30 seconds each   5 sets

Do each exercise for 30 seconds, recover for 30 seconds, then move on to the next exercise. Recover for 1 minute. Do the sets five times in total.

HIGH KNEE JOG (see page 157 for photos)

Set-up: Stand with your feet hip-width apart, knees slightly bent, and arms by your sides.

Action: Bring your left knee up to hip level, push off your right foot and switch legs, bringing your right leg up to hip level and landing on your left foot.

JESSIE'S TIP *Pump your arms as if you are running, and always land with your knees slightly bent.*

SPEED SKATE (see page 154 for photos)

Set-up: Stand with feet hip-width apart, knees slightly bent.

Action: Leap or step to the left side and land on your left leg, reach across with your right hand towards your left knee or toes. Repeat on the other side.

MOUNTAIN CLIMBERS

Set-up: Assume a press-up position, arms extended, hands on the floor, legs extended.

Action: Keeping your body in a straight line, bring your right knee towards your chest. Return to start and repeat with your left leg.

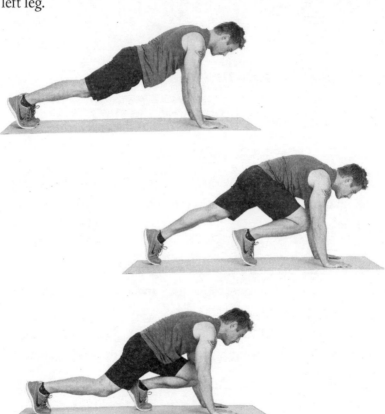

SWITCH JUMP LUNGES (see opposite above)

Set-up: Stand with feet shoulder-width apart, arms by your sides. Lunge forward with your right thigh parallel to the floor, left leg back.

Action: Jump up and switch leg positions. Land in a lunge with your left foot forward. Repeat on the other side.

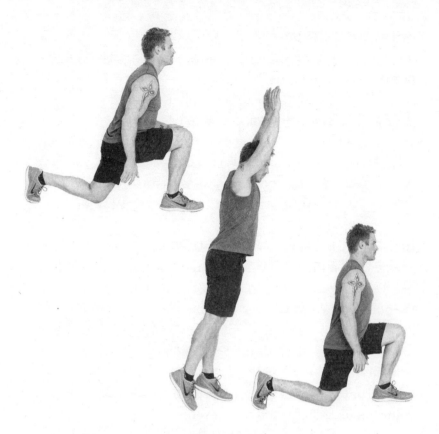

Day 8 BUILD: Strength training

Pull day

6 exercises   10 reps   4 sets

Perform each exercise ten times, and then move on to the next exercise. Recover for 30–60 seconds between sets.

BENT-OVER ROW (see Dumb-bell row, page 178 for photos)
Set-up: Stand with your feet hip-width apart, holding a dumb-bell in each hand, palms facing each other. Bend your knees slightly and bring your torso forward by bending at the waist. Keep your back long and almost parallel to the floor.

Action: Lift the dumb-bells to your sides until they pass your torso, keeping the dumb-bells close to your body. Lower to start position.

BICEPS CURLS (see page 179 for photos)
Set-up: Stand with feet shoulder-width apart, arms down by your sides, holding a dumb-bell in each hand, palms facing forwards.
Action: Keeping your elbows close to your torso, curl the dumb-bells up towards your shoulders. Lower to start position.

RESISTANCE BAND LAT PULL-DOWN
Set-up: Attach the resistance band door attachment to the top of a door. Face the door and hold both handles. Back away from the door until your arms are straight.
Action: With your feet hip-width apart and knees slightly bent, lower your torso towards the floor and extend your arms past your head. Pull the handles towards you until they are taut; bend your elbows out to the sides until your hands are next to your shoulders. Return to start position.

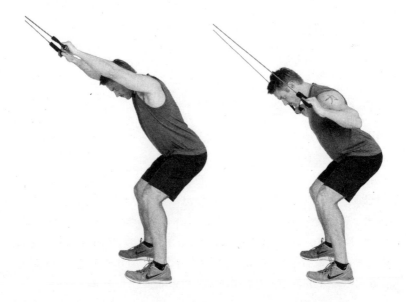

RESISTANCE BAND BICEPS CURLS

Set-up: Stand with both feet on the resistance band, feet shoulder-width apart, holding a handle in each hand.

Action: Keeping your elbows close to your torso, curl the handles up towards your shoulders. Slowly lower the band and repeat.

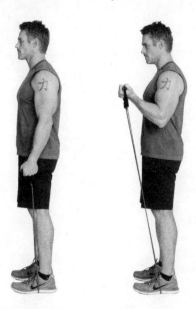

Day 9 BURN: Metabolic training

5 exercises   1 minute each   4 sets

Perform each exercise for 60 seconds, then move on to the next exercise. Complete one set, recover for 90 seconds. Do the sets four times in total.

SUMO SQUAT WITH DUMB-BELL 'SET IT DOWN, PICK IT UP' (see photos overleaf)

Set-up: Stand with your feet slightly wider than hip-width apart, toes pointing out, holding a dumb-bell with both hands at your chest.

Action: Bend your knees and lower your body until your thighs are parallel to the floor. Set the dumb-bell on the floor and push yourself back up to standing. Squat down again and pick up the dumb-bell.

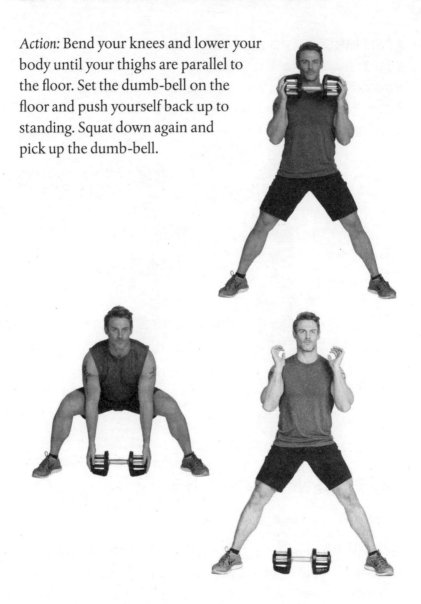

STABILITY BALL PRESS-UPS (see opposite above)
Set-up: Come into a plank position, with your toes or shins resting on the ball. Place your hands shoulder-width apart.
Action: Bend your elbows to a 90-degree angle then press back to starting position.

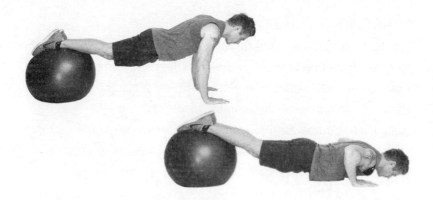

BENCH JUMP UP AND OVER

Set-up: Stand to the side of your bench with your left foot on the bench, and your right foot on the floor.
Action: Bend both knees and push off your right foot, jumping over to the left and landing with your right foot on the bench. Continue, alternating legs.

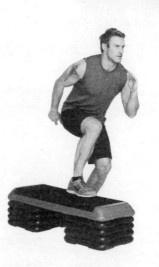

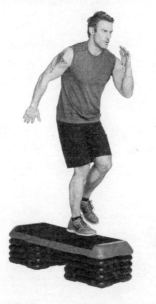

LUNGE WITH SINGLE-ARM ROW

Set-up: Hold a dumb-bell in your right hand, step your left leg forward and bend your left knee to 90 degrees. Lower your torso towards your left knee and place your left forearm on your left thigh. Push the dumb-bell towards the floor.

Action: Row the dumb-bell straight until your right elbow passes your torso. Return to starting position. Repeat for 30 seconds on the right side, then switch for 30 seconds on your left side.

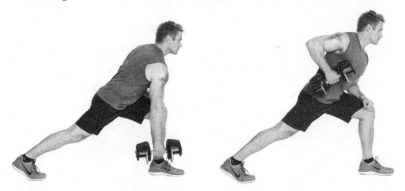

OPPOSITE TOE TOUCH CRUNCH

Set-up: Lie on your back with your legs extended. Place your right hand on the floor.

Action: Lift your upper body off the floor as you reach your left arm up and across to your right toes. Return to starting position. Complete all reps on right side then switch sides.

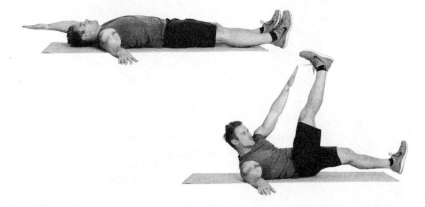

Day 10 BUILD: Strength training

Leg day

8 exercises   10 reps   4 sets

Perform each exercise ten times, and then move on to the next exercise. Recover for 30–60 seconds between sets.

DUMB-BELL GOBLET SQUAT

Set-up: Stand with feet shoulder-width apart. Hold a dumb-bell with both hands at chest level.

Action: Lower down into the bottom of a squat position. Keeping your heels pressing down into the floor, your back long and chest upright, push yourself back up to standing.

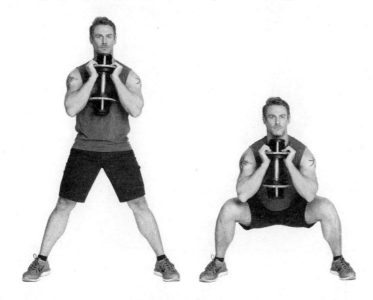

DEAD LIFT (see page 107 for photos)

Set-up: Stand with feet shoulder-width apart, toes pointing straight ahead. Hold a pair of dumb-bells in front of your thighs, palms facing your body.

Action: Keeping your back straight, hinge forward at your hips and lower your torso until it's almost parallel to the floor, lowering the dumb-bells towards your feet. Contract your hamstrings and glutes and push your hips forward to return to standing.

DUMB-BELL STEP-UP

Set-up: Stand with feet hip-width apart in front of a bench. Hold a dumb-bell in each hand with your arms by your sides.
Action: Place your right foot firmly on the bench. Push through your right heel to raise your body onto the bench, tap your left foot to the top of the bench and return to starting position.

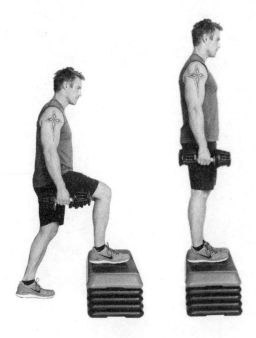

SPLIT SQUAT OFF BENCH (BULGARIAN SQUAT)

Set-up: Stand about 1m (3ft) in front of a bench, facing away from it. Hold a pair of dumb-bells by your sides. Put your right foot on top of the bench and shift your weight to your left foot.
Action: Bend your right knee and lower your body towards the

floor, keeping your left knee over your left ankle and bringing your left thigh parallel to the floor. Slowly stand back up to starting position.

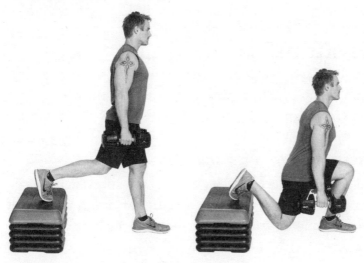

GLUTE BRIDGE ON BENCH

Set-up: Lie on the floor with your feet on the bench, knees bent to 90 degrees, arms by your sides.

Action: Press through your heels and lift your hips up, squeezing your glutes at the top. Slowly return to starting position.

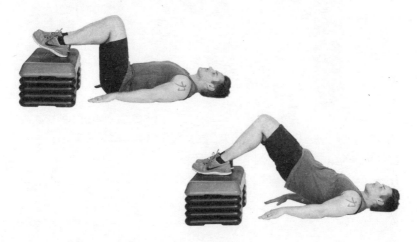

Day 11 BURN: Athletic training

HIIT athletic training

4 exercises   30 seconds each   5 sets

Do each exercise for 30 seconds, recover for 30 seconds, then move on to the next exercise.

Recover for 1 minute, then repeat the set. Do the sets five times in total.

JUMP FORWARD, JOG BACK

Set-up: Stand with feet shoulder-width apart, knees slightly bent. *Action:* Imagine there is a cone 1m (3ft) in front of you. Squat down and jump forward towards the cone. Jog back to starting position.

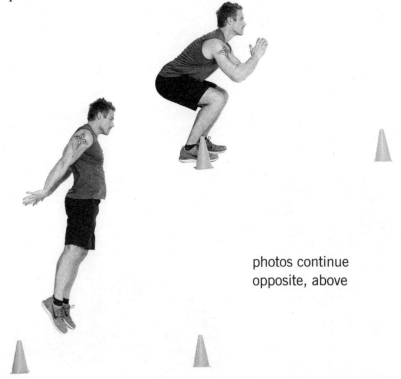

photos continue
opposite, above

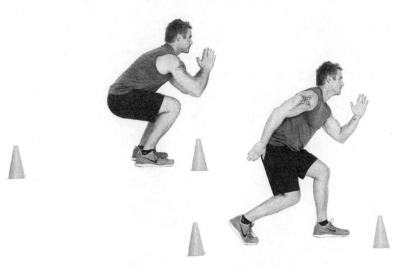

LUNGE KICK LUNGE (see page 177 for photos)
Set-up: Stand with feet shoulder-width apart, knees slightly bent.
Action: Step back with your right foot into a lunge, press off the ball of your right foot and kick your right leg forward. Repeat for 30 seconds, switching sides on the next circuit.

JESSIE'S TIP *Don't worry about how high you kick, focus on your balance and keeping your core engaged.*

PLANK JACKS
Set-up: Assume a press-up position: arms extended, palms on the floor, legs extended with feet together.
Action: Jump your feet out to the sides, and then back together.

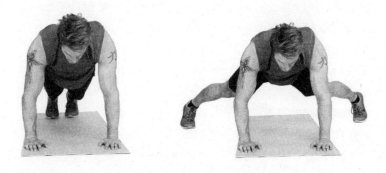

SQUAT JUMPS

Set-up: Stand with your feet shoulder-width apart, arms by your sides. Sit back into a squat until your thighs are parallel to the floor.

Action: Jump up explosively. Land with bent knees.

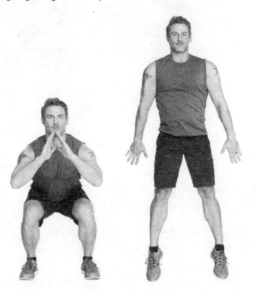

Day 12 BUILD: Strength training

Full body

5 exercises   10 reps   4 sets

Perform each exercise ten times, and then move on to the next exercise. Recover for 30–60 seconds between sets.

SIDE STEP-UP SHOULDER PRESS FRONT KICK

Set-up: Stand with your left side next to a bench, holding a dumb-bell in your left hand, elbow bent and palm facing in. Place your left foot on the step and bend your left knee.

Action: Straighten your left knee as you lift your right leg in

front of you and raise your left arm. Return
to starting position. Complete all reps on
the left side then switch sides.

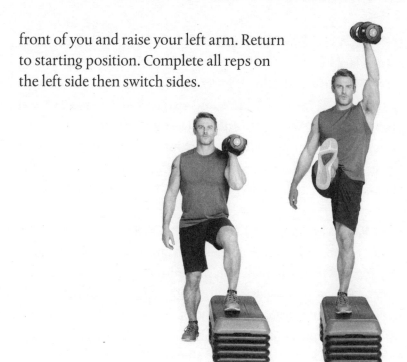

PLANK TO SIDE PLANK

Set-up: Get into a forearm plank position.

Action: Keeping your body straight, transfer your weight to your
left forearm and rotate your right arm towards the ceiling. Hold
side plank for one breath. Return to forearm plank. (10 reps is 5
planks on the right side and 5 planks on the left side)

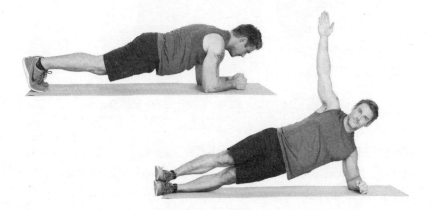

LUNGE WITH SINGLE-ARM ROW (see page 206 for photos)

Set-up: Hold a dumb-bell in your right hand, step your left leg forwards and bend your left knee to 90 degrees. Lower your torso towards your left knee and place your left forearm on your left thigh. Push the dumb-bell towards the floor.

Action: Pull the dumb-bell up until your right elbow passes your torso. Return to starting position. Repeat for 30 seconds on the right side, then switch for 30 seconds on your left side.

FORWARD LUNGES WITH BICEPS CURL

Set-up: Stand with your feet hip-width apart, arms by your sides, holding a dumb-bell in each hand, palms facing in.

Action: Take a step forward with your left foot and bend your left knee to 90 degrees, simultaneously curling the dumb-bells up towards your shoulders. Push off your left foot and return to starting position. Complete all reps on the left side then switch sides.

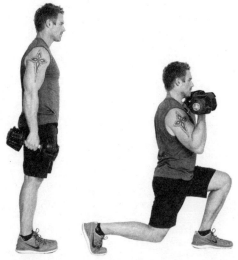

OPPOSITE TOE TOUCH CRUNCH (see page 206 for photos)

Set-up: Lie on your back with your legs extended. Place your right hand on the floor.

Action: Lift your upper body off the floor as you reach your left arm up and across to your right toes. Return to starting position. Complete all reps on the right side then switch sides.

Day 13: Slow Burn and Flow

Slow Burn

You should alternate walking with jogging at a very comfortable pace for 30 minutes.

Start by walking for a few minutes, then jog at a pace such that you could still have a conversation with someone. When you feel like you're working too hard to do that, or even if you're noticing that you're breathing heavily, slow down to a walk and keep walking until you feel completely recovered. You might alternate between walking and jogging four times each in 30 minutes, or even 10 times – anything is fine.

If you can, jog continuously for 30 minutes. You are not sprinting, so don't worry about your pace at all. You just want a comfortable, easy jog on relatively flat terrain.

If you feel breathless after 10 or 15 minutes, slow down to a brisk walk until you are completely recovered.

Flow

The Flow exercise routine for Day 13 is the same sequence that you first performed on Day 4, so simply repeat that – see page 159 for instructions and photos.

DAYS 14 TO 21

During these days you repeat the sequences carried out on earlier days, as follows:

Day 14: repeat Day 6   (see page 196)

Day 15: repeat Day 7   (see page 199)

Day 16: repeat Day 8   (see page 201)

Day 17: repeat Day 5   (see page 192)

Day 18: repeat Day 10   (see page 207)

Day 19: repeat Day 11   (see page 210)

Day 20: repeat Day 12   (see page 212)

Day 21: repeat Day 9   (see page 203)

ADVANCED WORKOUTS

Wake-Up workout

Starting on Day 5, do the following 4-minute circuit every day, to get you ready and energised for a healthy day. Do each exercise for 20 seconds, recover for 10 seconds and then move on to the next exercise. Do the circuit twice.

Advanced

Jumping Jacks	Press-ups
Squat Thrusts	Switch Jump Lunges

JUMPING JACKS (see page 168 for photos)
Set-up: Stand with your arms by your sides.
Action: Jump your legs out to the sides as you bring your arms overhead. Jump your feet back together and return arms to your sides.

SQUAT THRUSTS (see page 156 for photos)
Set-up: Stand with your feet together, arms by your sides.
Action: Bend your knees and place your palms on the floor with your arms on the outside of your knees; shift your weight onto your palms. Jump both feet back and land in plank position. Jump both feet forward and return to standing.

PRESS-UPS (see page 147 for photos)
Set-up: Lie on the floor on your stomach, with your hands close to your chest and your elbows at a 45-degree angle.
Action: Raise yourself off the floor until your arms are fully extended; your hands and the balls of your feet should support your weight. Keep a straight line from your head to your heels, contracting your abdominals and glutes so that your hips don't sag. Lower your chest to the floor and repeat.

SWITCH JUMP LUNGES (see page 201 for photos)

Set-up: Stand with feet shoulder-width apart, arms by your sides. Lunge forward with your right thigh parallel to the floor, your left leg back.

Action: Jump up and switch leg positions. Land in a lunge with your left foot forward. Repeat on the other side.

Day 5 BURN: Metabolic training

5 exercises   1 minute each   4 sets

Perform each exercise for 60 seconds, and then move on to the next exercise. Complete one set and recover for 90 seconds. Do the sets four times in total.

RENEGADE ROWS

Set-up: Assume the press-up position with your arms straight, feet slightly wider than shoulder-width and hands holding a pair of dumb-bells directly under your shoulders.

Action: Lift your right elbow towards the ceiling until your elbow passes your torso. Lower the weight and repeat on the other side.

SQUAT JUMPS (see page 212 for photos)

Set-up: Stand with feet shoulder-width apart, arms by your sides. Sit back into a squat until your thighs are parallel.

Action: Jump up explosively. Land with bent knees.

STABILITY BALL PRESS-UPS AND PIKES
(see pages 205 and 166 for photos)

Set-up: Start with your torso on the ball and hands and feet on the floor. Walk your hands forward until your legs are straight and your toes are on top of the ball. Hands are under shoulders.
Action: Lower your body until your chest almost touches the floor. Press your upper body back to starting position, keeping your legs straight; pull your feet towards your chest, pike your hips towards the ceiling as the ball rolls in, continue until your hips are directly under your shoulders. Slowly lower back to starting position. Continue alternating one press-up and one pike.

JUMP FORWARD, JOG BACK (see page 210 for photos)

Set-up: Stand with feet shoulder-width apart, and with knees slightly bent.
Action: Imagine a cone 1m (3 feet) in front of you. Squat down and jump forward towards the cone. Run back to starting position.

V-SIT WITH INCLINE DUMB-BELL CHEST PRESS

Set-up: Sit on the floor with your feet flat, holding a light dumb-bell in each hand in front of your shoulders. Lean back so that your torso is at a 45-degree angle.
Action: Engage your core and press the dumb-bells away from your body until your arms are straight. Return to start position.

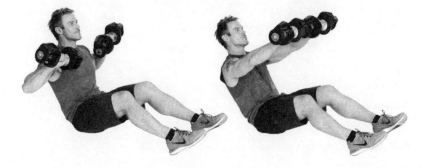

Day 6 BUILD: Strength training

Push day

5 exercises   15 reps   4 sets

Perform each exercise fifteen times, and then move on to the next exercise. Recover for 30–60 seconds between sets.

STABILITY BALL PRESS-UPS (see page 205 for photos)
Set-up: Come into a plank position, with your toes or shins resting on the ball, and your hands shoulder-width apart.
Action: Bend your elbows to a 90-degree angle, then press back to start position.

PISTOL SQUAT
Set-up: Stand on your left foot with your right leg extended in front of you.
Action: Bend your left knee and squat down as far as you can while keeping your right leg lifted. Extend your left leg to return to start position.

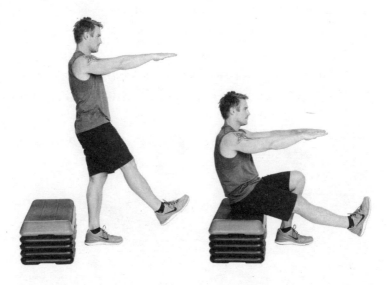

CHEST PRESS ON BENCH

Set-up: Lie on a bench holding a dumb-bell in each hand and your feet flat on the floor. Position the dumb-bells over your chest, with your palms facing forwards.

Action: Press the dumb-bells upwards above your chest, elbows straight but not locked. Lower the dumb-bells until they are level with your chest. Return to start position.

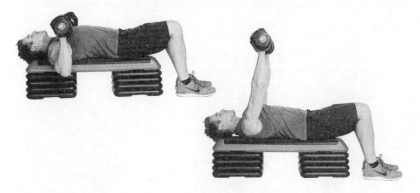

LYING TRICEPS EXTENSIONS ON BENCH

Set-up: Lie on a bench holding a dumb-bell in each hand. Extend your arms to a 90-degree angle from the floor.

Action: Bend your elbows so that your forearms are parallel to the floor. Straighten your arms without locking your elbows.

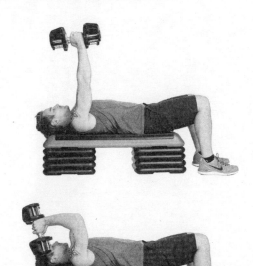

FRONT RAISE/LATERAL RAISE

Set-up: Stand with feet shoulder-width apart, holding a dumb-bell in each hand, palms facing your thighs.

Action: Keeping your elbows slightly bent, raise the dumb-bells in front of you until your arms are parallel to the floor. Lower to start position, turn your hands so palms face each other and raise the dumb-bells to the side until they are parallel to the floor. One front and one lateral raise are counted as one repetition.

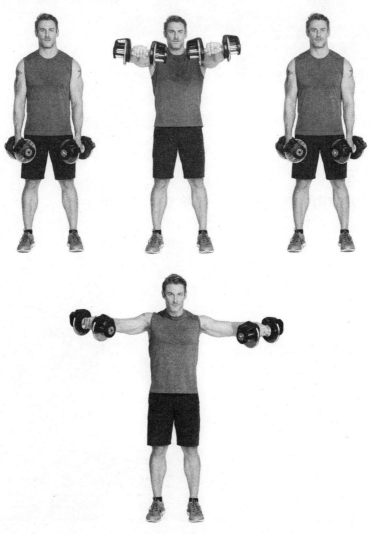

Day 7 BURN: Athletic training

Tabata training

7 exercises   20 seconds each   4 reps   1 set

Perform each exercise four times, working for 20 seconds then resting for 10 seconds. Recover for 30–60 seconds before moving on to the next exercise.

SPEED SKATE (see page 154 for photos)
Set-up: Stand with feet hip-width apart, knees slightly bent.
Action: Leap or step to the left side and land on your left leg, reach across with your right hand towards your left knee or toes. Repeat on the other side.

SPIDERMAN PUSH-UPS
Set-up: Start in a plank position with your hands under your shoulders.
Action: Bring your right knee outwards towards your right elbow. Return to start position and repeat with left leg.

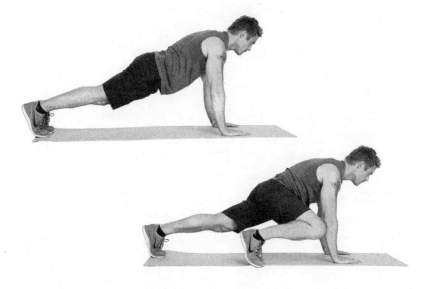

180-DEGREE JUMPS

Set-up: Stand with your feet hip-width apart and lower into a squat.

Action: Jump up, swinging your arms overhead and rotate yourself 180 degrees to the right while in the air. Land with knees bent and lower into a squat. Jump up, rotating 180 degrees to the left.

JESSIE'S TIP *If you aren't comfortable rotating 180 degrees, start with a 90-degree jump.*

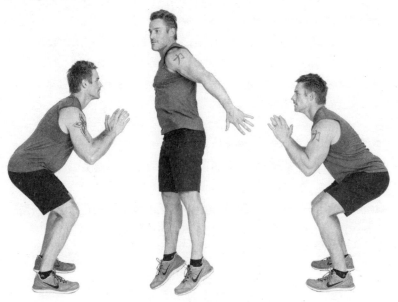

PLANK JACKS (see page 211 for photos)

Set-up: Start in a press-up position: arms extended, palms on the floor, and legs extended with feet together.

Action: Jump your feet out to the sides, and then back together.

SWITCH JUMP LUNGES (see page 201 for photos)

Set-up: Stand with feet shoulder-width apart, arms by your sides. Lunge forward with your right thigh parallel to the floor, left leg back.

Action: Jump up and switch leg positions. Land in a lunge with your left foot forward. Repeat on the other side.

RUSSIAN TWIST

Set-up: Sit on the floor with knees bent and heels about 30cm (12 inches) from your hips. Lean back slightly to a 45-degree angle without rounding your back.

Action: Place your arms in front of your chest, pull navel in to your spine and rotate torso to the right. Come back to centre and rotate left.

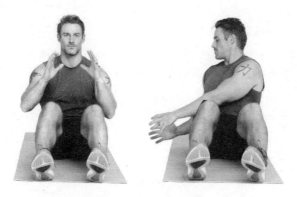

Day 8 BUILD: Strength training

Pull day

8 exercises   15 reps   4 sets

Perform each exercise fifteen times and then move on to the next exercise. Recover for 30–60 seconds between sets.

SINGLE-ARM ROW (see page 206 for photos)

Set-up: Stand in a staggered stance with your left foot forward and right leg back. Holding a dumb-bell in your right hand, bend at your hips and knees and lower your torso almost parallel to the floor. Extend your right arm.

Action: Pull the dumb-bell up until your elbow passes your torso, keeping elbow close to your side. Lower the dumb-bell back to start position.

BICEPS CURLS (see page 179 for photos)

Set-up: Stand with feet shoulder-width apart, arms down by your sides, holding a dumb-bell in each hand, palms facing forwards.

Action: Keeping your elbows close to your torso, curl the dumb-bells up towards your shoulders. Return to start position.

SINGLE-LEG DEAD LIFT

Set-up: Stand with your feet shoulder-width apart, toes pointing straight ahead. Hold a pair of dumb-bells in front of your thighs, with your palms facing your body.

Action: Lift your right leg a few inches off the floor, lower dumb-bells towards the floor as you raise your right leg behind you. Keep back straight and right knee slightly bent. Return to start position. Complete all reps on right side then switch sides.

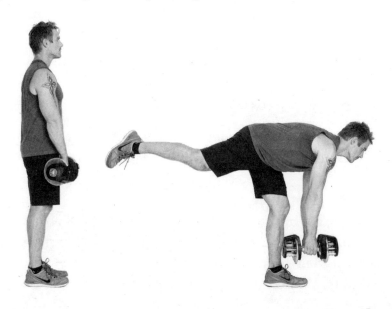

RESISTANCE BAND ROWS (see page 180 for photos)

Set-up: Attach the resistance band door attachment to chest height. Stand facing the door, holding both handles, with knees slightly bent.

Action: Reach forward with your arms in line with your shoulders. Pull the band back until your elbows pass your torso. Return to start position.

LAT PULLOVERS

Set-up: Lie on a bench or mat with knees bent, holding a dumb-bell in each hand over your chest, keeping your elbows slightly bent.

Action: Extend your arms over your chest, palms facing in. Keeping your elbows slightly bent, lower the dumb-bells in an arc back over your head, towards the floor. Bring your elbows level with your head, then return to start position.

JESSIE'S TIP *If you are using heavier weights, hold one heavy dumb-bell with both hands.*

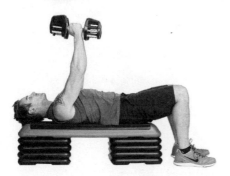

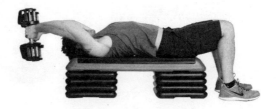

Day 9 BURN: Metabolic training

5 exercises   1 minute each   4 sets

Perform each exercise for 60 seconds, and then move on to the next exercise. Complete one set, recover for 90 seconds, then repeat. Do the sets four times in total.

STRADDLE BENCH JUMPS

Set-up: Stand on a bench with your knees slightly bent and your arms in front at shoulder height.

Action: Jump down to straddle the bench, landing in a squat, jump back onto the bench, landing with your feet together and knees bent.

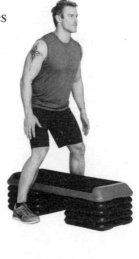

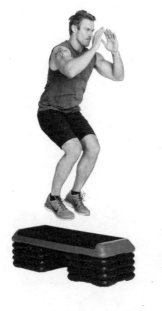

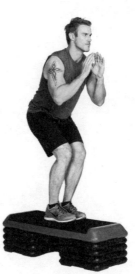

SINGLE-LEG DEAD LIFT WITH ROW

Set-up: Stand with feet shoulder-width apart, toes pointing straight ahead. Hold a pair of dumb-bells in front of your thighs, with your palms facing your body.

Action: Lift right leg a few inches off the floor, lower dumb-bells towards the floor as you raise your right leg behind you. Keep your back straight and left knee slightly bent. Pull the dumb-bells up towards your torso. Return to start position. Repeat for 30 seconds on the right side then switch sides.

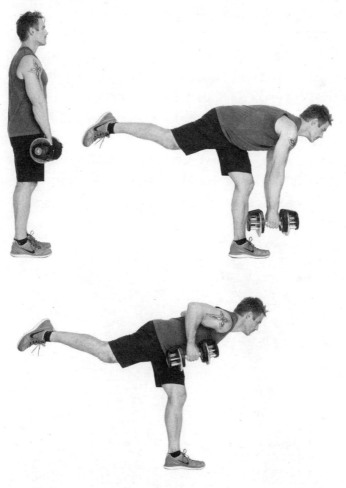

FORWARD LUNGES WITH BICEPS CURL

(see page 214 for photos)

Set-up: Stand with your feet hip-width apart, arms by your sides, holding a dumb-bell in each hand, palms facing in.

Action: Take a step forwards with your left foot and bend your right knee to 90 degrees, simultaneously curling the dumb-bells up towards your shoulders. Push off your left foot and return to start position. Complete all reps on left side then switch sides.

CURTSY, LUNGE, SQUAT ON BENCH

Set-up: Stand behind the narrow end of the bench with a dumb-bell in each hand. Step your left foot onto bench, step your right leg behind you and to the left so that your thighs cross, bend both knees and keep hips pointing forward.

Action: Press off your right foot and lunge behind the bench. Press off right foot again and step into a squat. Keeping your left foot on the bench, press down with your left foot to lift your right leg onto bench and raise your arms. Complete all reps on left side then switch sides.

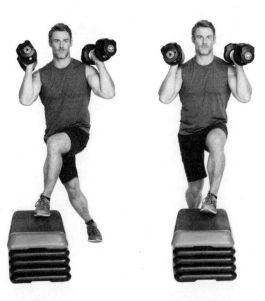

photos continue opposite, above

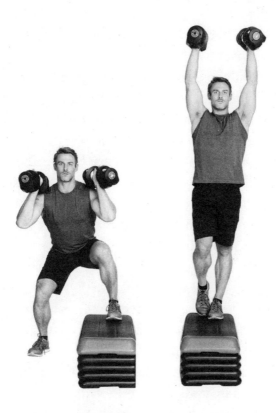

PLANK WITH KNEE CROSS (see page 192 for photos)
Set-up: Start in a plank position with your hands directly under your shoulders.
Action: Bring your right knee towards your left elbow. Return to start position and repeat with your left leg.

Day 10 BUILD: Strength training

Leg day

7 exercises   15 reps   4 sets

Perform each exercise fifteen times, and then move on to the next exercise. Recover for 30–60 seconds between sets.

CURTSY, LUNGE, SQUAT ON BENCH

(see page 230 for photos)

Set-up: Stand behind the narrow end of a bench with a dumb-bell in each hand. Step your left foot onto bench, step your right leg behind you and to the left so that your thighs cross, bend both knees and keep hips pointing forwards.

Action: Press off your right foot and lunge behind the bench. Press off your right foot again and step into a squat. Keeping your left foot on the bench, press down with your left foot to lift your right leg onto the bench and raise your arms. Repeat all reps on left side then switch sides.

DEAD LIFT (see page 107 for photos)

Set-up: Stand with your feet shoulder-width apart, toes point-ing straight ahead. Hold a pair of dumb-bells in front of your thighs, with palms facing your body.

Action: Keeping your back straight, hinge forward at your hips and lower your torso until it's almost parallel to the floor, lowering the dumb-bells towards your feet. Squeeze your glutes and push your hips forward to return to standing.

PISTOL SQUAT (see page 220 for photos)

Set-up: Stand on your left foot with left leg extended in front of you.

Action: Bend your left knee and squat down as far as you can while keeping right leg lifted. Extend your left leg to return to start position.

SINGLE LEG GLUTE BRIDGE ON BENCH

(see opposite above)

Set-up: Lie on the floor with your feet on the bench, knees bent to 90 degrees, arms by your sides.

Action: Press through your left heel and lift your right leg and

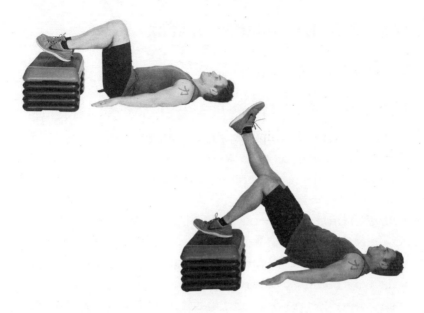

your hips up, squeezing your glutes at the top. Slowly return to start position.

PULSE SQUATS

Set-up: Stand with your feet hip-width apart, arms raised.
Action: Bend your knees as though you're sitting down in a chair until your thighs are nearly parallel to the floor. Hold the squat position and pulse a few inches up and down 15 times.

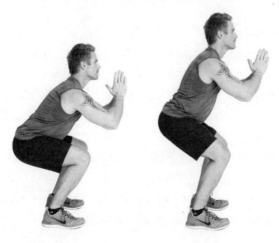

Day 11 BURN: Athletic training

Tabata training

6 exercises   20 seconds each   4 reps   1 set

Perform each exercise four times, working for 20 seconds, then resting for 10 seconds. Recover for 30–60 seconds before moving on to the next exercise.

SQUAT THRUSTS (see page 156 for photos)
Set-up: Stand with your feet together, arms by your sides.
Action: Bend your knees and place your palms on the floor with your arms on the outside of your knees; shift your weight onto your palms. Jump both feet back and land in plank position. Jump both feet forwards and return to standing.

JUMP FORWARD, JOG BACK (see page 210 for photos)
Set-up: Stand with your feet shoulder width apart, knees slightly bent.
Action: Imagine there is a cone 1m (3ft) in front of you. Squat down and jump forward towards the cone. Jog back to starting position

MOUNTAIN CLIMBERS (see page 200 for photos)
Set-up: Assume a press-up position, arms extended, hands on the floor, legs extended.
Action: Keeping your body in a straight line, bring your right knee towards your chest. Return to start and repeat with your left leg.

PASS THE BALL, SHOOT THE BALL (see page 153 for photos)
Set-up: Stand with your feet slightly wider than hip-width apart, knees slightly bent and hands at chest level.

Action: Imagine you are holding a football at your chest; pivot to your left side and push your arms out as if passing the ball. Come back to starting position and jump up or lift up on your toes and pretend to shoot the ball. Repeat on the other side.

PLANK WITH KNEE CROSS (see page 192 for photos)
Set-up: Start in a plank position with your hands under your shoulders.
Action: Bring your right knee towards your left elbow. Return to start position and repeat with your left leg.

HIGH KNEE JOG (see page 157 for photos)
Set-up: Stand with feet hip-width apart, knees slightly bent, and arms by your sides.
Action: Bring your left knee up to hip level, right arm reaching towards the ceiling; push off your right foot and switch legs and arms, bringing your right leg up to hip level and left arm towards the ceiling.

Day 12 BUILD: Strength training

Full body

6 exercises   15 reps   4 sets

Perform each exercise fifteen times and then move on to the next exercise. Recover for 30–60 seconds between sets.

RENEGADE ROWS (see page 218 for photos)
Set-up: Assume the press-up position with your arms straight, feet slightly wider than shoulder-width apart and hands holding a pair of dumb-bells directly under your shoulders.

Action: Lift your right elbow towards the ceiling until your elbow passes your torso. Lower the weight and repeat on the other side. Each row is counted as one rep.

LUNGE WITH OVERHEAD PRESS

Set-up: Stand with feet shoulder-width apart, holding a dumb-bell in each hand, arms by your sides, palms facing each other.
Action: Curl dumb-bells up to your shoulders as you step your left foot forward into a lunge. Press dumb-bells overhead, then press into your left heel to return to standing.

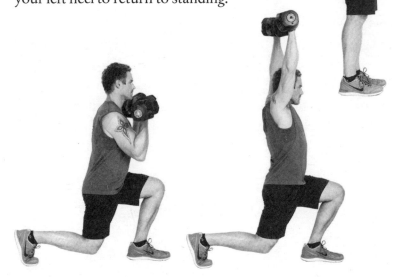

CHEST FLY LAT PULLOVER ON STABILITY BALL

Set-up: Sit on the stability ball holding a dumb-bell in each hand, dumb-bells resting on your thighs. Slowly walk your feet forward and slide your torso down the ball until your head, shoulders and upper back are on the ball. Your feet should be parallel and knees shoulder-width apart, bent 90 degrees so that your thighs and torso are parallel to the floor.

Action: Position the dumb-bells over your chest, palms facing each other. Press the dumb-bells upwards above your chest, elbows straight but not locked. Lower the dumb-bells until they are level with your chest. Press the dumb-bells back to starting position and lower the dumb-bells behind your head. Bring the dumb-bells over your chest. One rep is one chest fly and one lat pullover.

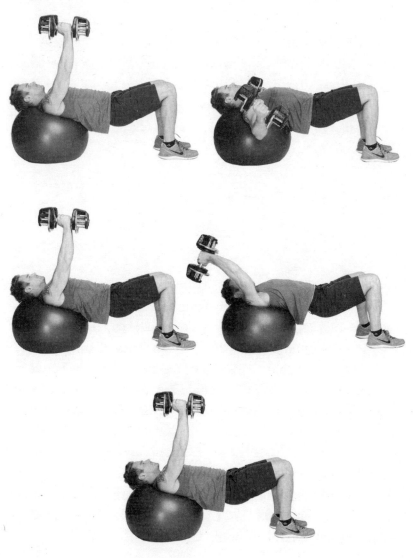

STABILITY BALL BACK EXTENSION (see page 167 for photos)
Set-up: Lie face down on a stability ball with your hands on the ball, about 15cm (6 inches) apart. Press your feet against a wall or sturdy object.
Action: Lift your torso up until your body forms a straight line.

JESSIE'S TIP *To make it more challenging, place your fingertips behind your head.*

SUMO SQUAT BICEPS CURL (see page 172 for photos)
Set-up: Stand with feet slightly wider than hip-width apart, toes out, holding a dumb-bell in each hand, palms facing in.
Action: Bend your knees and lower your body until your thighs are parallel to the floor. Push yourself back up as you curl the dumb-bells to your shoulders.

Day 13: Slow Burn and Flow

Slow Burn

Try to jog continuously for 30 minutes today. You are not sprinting, so don't worry about your pace at all. You want a comfortable, easy jog on relatively flat terrain. If you feel breathless after 10 or 15 minutes, slow down to a brisk walk until you are completely recovered, then resume jogging. Alternate between brisk walking and jogging at any point, as many times as you feel comfortable, but try to move continuously for 30 minutes.

Flow

The Flow exercise routine for Day 13 is the same sequence that you first performed on Day 4, so simply repeat that – see page 159 for instructions and photos.

DAYS 14 TO 21

During these days you repeat the sequences carried out on earlier days, as follows:

Day 14: repeat Day 6   (see page 220)

Day 15: repeat Day 7   (see page 223)

Day 16: repeat Day 8   (see page 225)

Day 17: repeat Day 5   (see page 218)

Day 18: repeat Day 10 (see page 231)

Day 19: repeat Day 11 (see page 234)

Day 20: repeat Day 12 (see page 235)

Day 21: repeat Day 9   (see page 228)

WEEKEND WARRIOR WORKOUT CHALLENGE

How many can you do? Challenge yourself by repeating exercises from each style of training (strength, athletic, metabolic) at your appropriate level, with more intensity and more repetitions than usual. Perform each exercise set once, recover for 30–60 seconds, then move on to the next exercise in the sequence. Once you have finished set 4, take a 2-minute break if you need it, then repeat the entire sequence as many times as you can (taking the 60-second rest between sets and the 2-minute break after the fourth set). Record your results and try it again when you are well rested next week and are up for a challenge!

Set 1

Strength training (push): Knee press-ups (page 148)

Athletic training: Pass the ball, shoot the ball (page 153)

Metabolic training: Squat with dumb-bell overhead press (page 195)

Set 2

Strength training (pull): Dumb-bell row (page 108)

Athletic training: Side shuffles (page 152)

Metabolic training: Alternating step-ups (page 171)

Set 3

Strength training (legs): Squats (page 106)

Athletic training: Lunge kick lunge (page 176)

Metabolic training: Sumo squat biceps curl (page 172)

Set 4

Strength training (full body): Squat knee raise (page 187)

Athletic training: Alternating elbow to knee (page 177)

Metabolic training: Reverse lunge lateral raise (page 172)

BONUS WEEKEND YOGA WORKOUT

Before the workout, take a moment to sit cross-legged. Let your thoughts go, release your 'to-do' list and anything you may have been stressed about lately. This is your time. This is your space. Take it and reap the benefits of a calmer, more energised day after your practice. Take five deep breaths. On the breath in, say silently, in your head, 'acceptance'. On the breath out, say 'peace'. Now move on to the postures.

STRETCH

Stand up and reach your arms high above your head, stretching your ribs up and taking two deep breaths. Bend over to your right, keeping your shoulders down even though your arms are above your head. Next, bend to your left, allowing your right side to stretch out and elongate. Come back to standing straight and drop your arms.

Now stretch your arms up once more and immediately bend forwards at the waist until you are hanging over your legs, only as deeply as your body wants to go. Make sure you release any tension in your head and neck. Let the tension melt off you like snow melting off a tree in the sun.

DOWNWARD-FACING DOG

Come into downward-facing dog (see page 159). You've prac-tised this pose as part of your Flow workout, but this time you are leaning down into it from the stretch, rather than rising into it from a plank. Bend your legs and plant your hands on the ground, shoulder-width apart. Keep your feet about shoulder-width apart, legs as straight as possible, and bring the hips up high while keeping your back straight and hingeing at the waist. Your palms are planted firmly on the ground. Your head and neck should be between your upper arms. Bend your knees as much as you need to while maintaining equal weight on your hands and feet. Hold for three to five breath cycles, releasing a little more tension on each breath out and sinking into the pose.

PLANK AND CHATURANGA HOLDS

Come into plank position (or the upper part of a push-up) and hold it for five breaths. Now, slowly lower yourself down, elbows tight against your body, without touching the floor, and hold, hovering like this, for one or two breaths. This lower press-up position is called 'chaturanga' in yoga. Next, release and lie on the floor on your stomach for two breaths. Now get back into upper plank position, hold for five breaths again, lower into chaturanga (that lower push-up position, ensuring your butt is low and in line with your shoulders as much as possible). Keep a straight back, just like a regular plank. It's not easy! This is a great core and arm and leg workout. Hold it for three breaths this time. Lower down and then do upward-facing dog (arch your back up, look up to the sky, shoulders dropped, and keep your hips and legs on the ground) for three to five breaths.

SIDE PLANKS

From the floor or standing, come into downward-facing dog. Now switch onto your right foot and right hand only, looking out to the side and holding side plank. Keep your body in a straight line. Hold for four breaths. Come back to downward-facing dog, and switch over to the other side-facing plank. Hold for four breaths. Keep your core tight through all poses and transitions – breathe while you move and hold!

Move back into downward-facing dog. Walk or jump your feet in until you're hanging over your legs, then 'roll up', one vertebra at a time, to standing. Ground your feet into the floor and shake off any tension.

CHAIR POSE

Squat, while sticking your butt out, holding your back and neck long and straight, until you are in chair pose. Reach your arms over your head parallel to your shoulders. Reach, even as you hold your squat. Stay in this position for five breaths. Come to standing.

SQUAT WORK

Take 15 deep squats with your hands on your hips and straighten while breathing deeply. At the top (when you're standing tall), squeeze your butt and at the low point of the squat (when you're sitting) stick your butt out like you're sitting on a chair. Keep your back straight, core tight, shoulders dropped. You'll feel this in your glutes!

TREE BALANCE POSE

Bring one foot up until the flat of your foot is against the inside of your standing leg. Stand straight and balance on one foot by engaging your core. Lift your hands above your head and touch your palms together. Hold as long as you can! Can you hold it for about six breaths? Breathe deeply. You are learning to stay balanced, while clearing your mind and strengthening your core muscles.

CLOSING MEDITATION

Come back to standing, bring your hands together in prayer in front of your chest.

Take some deep breaths with your eyes closed, simply do nothing and feel your breath in your body as you learn to be present and accept yourself. Next, silently thank yourself for taking this time to honour your body and health. Sending gratitude to your body and self will increase your acceptance and help strengthen your resolve to make healthy choices for your diet, exercise and life.

CHAPTER 8

THE RECIPES

··

I'm a pretty basic cook, so most of the recipes that follow are basic too. The food exchange lists and the nutrition information provided in the meal plan day charts can help you make swaps from meal to meal if you feel like making something different but want to stick to your PCF ratio. If you want to follow the meal plan strictly, most meals have a recipe provided, but the snacks and a few of the dinners are so straightforward as not to need one (I assume you already have your own preferred method of grilling steak or poaching salmon, for example).

Many people find that as they move more, they are hungrier and food simply tastes better. Take advantage of this if it happens to you on The Programme, and use the opportunity to find new ingredients you love and healthy foods that make you feel great.

A FEW TIPS

Cooking spray is a great addition to your store cupboard. It prevents sticking and saves calories by giving a very light, even coating of oil to pans.

Measuring spoons It would be a good idea to buy a set of measuring spoons. The spoons you use in your kitchen may be bigger or smaller than the standard teaspoons (5ml) and tablespoons (15ml) that are used to measure ingredients.

Digital temperature probe If you are worried about cooking chicken and turkey thoroughly, you might want to invest in a temperature probe. This is a spike attached to a thermometer: push the spike into the centre of the food and check the reading. But it's not difficult to test when meat or poultry is cooked: simply insert a thin skewer, and if the juices run clear or golden (not pink) then the food is cooked.

All recipes serve 1 person, except where otherwise stated.

SMOOTHIES

You can use whatever type of protein powder you prefer in the smoothies. I recommend whey-, pea-, or hemp-based powders as a first choice. Packs of protein powder come with a scoop that usually holds 30g (1oz) – check the pack in case your scoop is a different size – and fill it level (not rounded).

Green Tea Smoothie   CLEANSE DAYS

240ml (9fl oz) brewed green tea, cooled
1 scoop protein powder
½ medium banana
1 tbsp lemon juice
1 tbsp ground flaxseed (linseed)
30g (1oz) fresh spinach leaves

Put all the ingredients into a blender, add ice to taste and blend until smooth.

Nutrition: 200 calories, 4g fat (1g saturated fat), 20g carbs (9g sugar), 4g fibre, 24g protein
Exchanges: 3 protein, 1 fruit, 1 vegetable, 1 fat

Upgraded Green Tea Smoothie

BURN OR BUILD DAYS

240ml (9fl oz) brewed green tea, cooled
1 scoop protein powder
1 medium banana
1 tbsp lemon juice
2 tbsp ground flaxseed (linseed)
30g (1oz) fresh spinach leaves

Put all the ingredients into a blender, add ice to taste and blend until smooth.

Nutrition: 290 calories, 7g fat (1g saturated fat), 36g carbs (16g sugar), 8g fibre, 26g protein
Exchanges: 3 protein, 2 fruits, ½ vegetable, 2 fats

Chocolate-Covered Strawberry Smoothie CLEANSE DAYS

240ml (9fl oz) plain unsweetened almond milk
1 scoop protein powder
2 tbsp unsweetened cocoa powder
175g (6oz) strawberries, sliced

Put all the ingredients into a blender, add ice to taste and blend until smooth.

Nutrition 214 calories, 5g fat (1g saturated fat), 25g carbs (10g sugar), 9g fibre, 21g protein
Exchanges 3 protein, 1 fruit, 1 fat

Upgraded Chocolate-Covered Strawberry Smoothie BURN OR BUILD DAYS

240ml (9fl oz) plain unsweetened almond milk
1 scoop protein powder
2 tbsp unsweetened cocoa powder
325g (11½oz) strawberries, sliced
1 tbsp chia seeds
1 tbsp dark chocolate chips (at least 70% cocoa solids)

Put all the ingredients into a blender, add ice to taste and blend until smooth.

Nutrition 370 calories, 14g fat (4g saturated fat), 45g carbs (25g sugar), 15g fibre, 25g protein
Exchanges 3 protein, 2 fruits, 2 fats

Java Mocha Smoothie CLEANSE DAYS

240ml (9fl oz) brewed coffee, cooled
175g (6oz) fat-free plain Greek yogurt
1 tbsp unsweetened cocoa powder
½ medium banana
1 tbsp ground flaxseed (linseed)

Put all the ingredients into a blender, add ice to taste and blend until smooth.

Nutrition 192 calories, 4g fat (0.5g saturated fat), 25g carbs (13g sugar), 6g fibre, 21g protein
Exchanges 1 dairy, ½ fruit, 1 fat

Upgraded Java Mocha Smoothie

BURN OR BUILD DAYS

240ml (9fl oz) brewed coffee, cooled
250g (9oz) fat-free plain Greek yogurt
1 tbsp unsweetened cocoa powder
2 tbsp ground flaxseed (linseed)
1 medium banana

Put all the ingredients into a blender, add ice to taste and blend until smooth.

Nutrition 310 calories, 6g fat (0.5g saturated fat), 44g carbs (24g sugar), 9g fibre, 26g protein
Exchanges 1+ dairy, 2 protein, 2 fruits, 2 fats

Tropical Kale Smoothie CLEANSE DAYS

175g (6oz) fat-free plain Greek yogurt
120ml (4fl oz) water
85g (3oz) chopped pineapple
1 tbsp ground flaxseed (linseed)
75g (2½oz) chopped kale

Put all the ingredients into a blender, add ice to taste and blend until smooth.

Nutrition: 200 calories, 3g fat (0g saturated fat), 27g carbs (15g sugar), 4g fibre, 22g protein
Exchanges: 1 dairy, 1 fruit, ½ vegetable, 1 fat

Upgraded Tropical Kale Smoothie

BURN OR BUILD DAYS

250g (9oz) fat-free plain Greek yogurt
120ml (4fl oz) water
175g (6oz) chopped pineapple
1 tbsp ground flaxseed (linseed)
100g (3½oz) chopped kale

Put all the ingredients into a blender, add ice to taste and blend until smooth.

Nutrition: 290 calories, 4g fat (0g saturated fat), 43g carbs (24g sugar), 6g fibre, 27g protein
Exchanges: 1+ dairy, 2 fruits, 1½ vegetables, 1 fat

Cherry Almond Smoothie CLEANSE DAYS

240ml (9fl oz) unsweetened plain almond milk
200g (7oz) unsweetened frozen cherries
1 scoop protein powder
30g (1oz) fresh spinach leaves (optional)

Put all the ingredients into a blender and blend until smooth.

Nutrition: 220 calories, 4.5g fat (1g saturated fat), 23g carbs (14g sugar),
4g fibre, 24g protein
Exchanges: 3 protein, 1 fruit, ½ vegetable, 1 fat

Upgraded Cherry Almond Smoothie
BURN OR BUILD DAYS

240ml (9fl oz) unsweetened almond milk
400g (14oz) unsweetened frozen cherries
1 scoop protein powder
40g (1½oz) fresh spinach leaves (optional)
1 tbsp ground flaxseed (linseed)

Put all the ingredients into a blender and blend until smooth.

Nutrition: 330 calories, 7g fat (1g saturated fat), 44g carbs (28g sugar),
9g fibre, 26g protein
Exchanges: 3 protein, 2 fruits, 1 vegetable, 2 fats

Blueberry Pear Smoothie CLEANSE DAYS

240ml (9fl oz) unsweetened fat-free kefir (see page 58)
50g (1¾oz) blueberries
50g (1¾oz) chopped ripe pear
1 tbsp chia seeds
20g (¾oz) rocket (optional)

Put all the ingredients into a blender and blend until smooth.

Nutrition: 211 calories, 3g fat (1g saturated fat), 32g carbs (22g sugar), 8g fibre, 15g protein
Exchanges: 1 dairy, 1 fruit, ½ vegetable, 1 fat

Upgraded Blueberry Pear Smoothie

BURN OR BUILD DAYS

240ml (9fl oz) unsweetened fat-free kefir (see page 58)
75g (2½oz) blueberries
100g (3½oz) chopped ripe pear
1 tbsp chia seeds
30g (1oz) rocket (optional)
½ scoop protein powder

Put all the ingredients into a blender and blend until smooth.

Nutrition: 320 calories, 4.5g fat (1g saturated fat), 46g carbs (28g sugar), 10g fibre, 31g protein
Exchanges: 1 dairy, 1 protein, 2 fruits, 1 vegetable, 1 fat

SOUPS

Vegetable Stock

This makes a good base for other soups. You can also sip a cup of hot stock as a warming snack at any time on The Programme.

MAKES 3.5 LITRES (6 pints)

3.8 litres (6½ pints) water
1 large onion, chopped
1 head of celery, chopped
6 garlic cloves, peeled and halved
6 sprigs of thyme
1 bunch of parsley stems
2 bay leaves
1 tsp sea salt
1 tsp black peppercorns

Put all the ingredients into a large pan and simmer for 1 hour. Strain through a fine mesh strainer into a large bowl and cool before storing in the refrigerator or freezer.

Exchanges You can use the vegetable stock as a 'free' food to eat whenever you wish.

Carrot and Ginger Soup CLEANSE DAY

If you are not eating this during a Cleanse day, it would be delicious with the addition of a little seafood, such as seared scallops.

SERVES 8; approximately 350ml (12fl oz) per serving

1 tbsp olive oil
½ onion, chopped
2 garlic cloves, crushed
85g (3oz) fresh ginger, peeled and sliced
1 tsp ground cumin
1.3kg (3lb) carrots, chopped
1.7 litres (3 pints) vegetable stock
sea salt and ground white pepper
100g (3½oz) broccoli florets, broken into very small florets
3 tbsp chopped fresh chives

In a large saucepan, heat the olive oil and sweat the onion, garlic, ginger and cumin for 5 minutes. Add the carrots and cook for an additional 5 minutes. Pour in the stock and simmer until the carrots are tender.

Transfer to a blender and blend until smooth, adding salt and pepper to taste, then, if you wish, pass through a fine mesh strainer. Blanch the broccoli in boiling water for 5 minutes until bright green and stir into the soup. Serve sprinkled with chopped chives.

Nutrition 128 calories, 2.5g fat, 25g carbs (9g sugar), 6g fibre, 2g protein
Exchanges 3 vegetables, ½ fat

White Bean and Tuscan Kale Soup

CLEANSE DAYS

This soup is even tastier with a spoonful of Rocket Pesto (see overleaf) as a garnish.

SERVES 8; approximately 350ml (12fl oz) per serving

600g (1lb 5oz) dried white beans, soaked overnight
1 tbsp olive oil
½ onion, cut into small dice
3 garlic cloves, finely chopped
5 carrots, diced
1 tbsp chopped flat-leaf parsley
1 tsp chopped thyme
½ tsp chopped rosemary
1.7 litres (3 pints) vegetable stock
1 bay leaf
1 tbsp sea salt
85g (3oz) cavolo nero or kale, shredded
Rocket Pesto (see below)

Drain the beans and cook in water for approximately 1 hour, or until al dente. Drain them and set aside.

In a large saucepan, heat the olive oil and sweat the onion, garlic, carrots and herbs for 5 minutes. Add the stock, bay leaf and salt and simmer until the carrots are tender. Remove from the heat and remove the bay leaf. Add the beans and kale and stir the soup until the kale is bright green and just tender. Serve hot, with 1 tsp rocket pesto in each bowl of soup. If you are not serving immediately, allow to cool and store in the refrigerator.

Nutrition 160 calories, 2g fat, 28g carbs (6g sugar), 7g fibre, 8g protein
Exchanges 1 starch, 1 protein, 2+ vegetables, ½ fat

Rocket Pesto Garnish

175g (6oz) wild rocket
½ tbsp toasted pine nuts
1 garlic clove, peeled
juice of ½ lemon
½ tsp sea salt
3 tbsp olive oil

Put all the ingredients – except the olive oil – into a food processor or blender. Blend until combined, then slowly add the oil until the pesto is thick and emulsified.

Nutrition (1 tsp of pesto): 25 calories, 2.5g fat
Exchanges: ½ fat

Curried Cauliflower Soup CLEANSE

For additional protein on non-cleanse days, add seafood such as prawns.

SERVES 8 (approximately 350ml/12fl oz per serving)

1 tbsp olive oil
2 cauliflowers, roughly chopped (reserve some small florets for garnish)
6 garlic cloves, sliced
1 large onion, chopped
1½ tbsp curry powder
120ml (4fl oz) coconut milk
1 litre (1¾ pints) vegetable stock
sea salt to taste

GARNISH

1 tbsp small cauliflower florets
1 tsp olive oil
2 tsp sultanas
1 tsp toasted pine nuts
½ tsp chopped parsley
½ tsp grated lemon zest
sea salt to taste

In a large saucepan, heat the olive oil and sauté the cauliflower, garlic, onion and curry powder over medium heat until the cauliflower starts to become tender.

Add the coconut milk and stir to loosen the residue from the bottom of the pan. Simmer for 3 minutes, then add the stock and simmer for about 30 minutes.

Transfer to a blender and blend until smooth, adding salt to taste, then pass through a fine mesh strainer.

For the garnish: sauté the cauliflower florets in the oil over medium heat until evenly golden brown. Turn off the heat and add the sultanas, pine nuts, parsley and lemon zest, and season with a pinch of salt.

Gently reheat the soup if necessary and sprinkle with the garnish.

Nutrition: 103 calories, 6g fat (3.5g saturated fat), 11g carbs (5g sugar), 4g fibre, 3.5g protein
Exchanges: 2 vegetables, 1 fat

Tomato-Cucumber Gazpacho

CLEANSE DAYS

This chilled soup is best if you make it the day before you want to eat it. For additional protein on non-Cleanse days, serve with seafood such as grilled prawns, scallops or salmon.

SERVES 6; approximately 500ml (18fl oz) per serving

2 × 400g cans good quality plum tomatoes in juice, chopped and juice reserved
1½ cucumbers, peeled and cut into small dice
¼ red onion, cut into small dice
1 bunch of spring onions, tops only, finely chopped
½ bunch of coriander, finely chopped
4 tbsp rice wine vinegar
1 tbsp Tabasco sauce
juice of 1 lemon
3 tsp sea salt
1 avocado, ripe but firm, cut into small dice
30g (1oz) watercress leaves

Put all the ingredients, except half the lemon juice, the avocado and the watercress, into a large mixing bowl and stir to combine. Add the avocado and mix gently. Taste and adjust the seasoning if necessary and add as much juice as you wish to reach the desired consistency. Leave to marinate overnight in the refrigerator for the best results. Before serving, toss the watercress with the reserved lemon juice and use to garnish the gazpacho. Serve cold.

Nutrition: 92 calories, 4g fat, 12g carbs (7g sugar), 5g fibre, 3g protein
Exchanges: 2 vegetables, 1 fat

Mushroom and Pak Choi Soup

CLEANSE DAYS

For additional protein on non-Cleanse days, serve with shredded chicken or lentils.

SERVES 6 (approximately 500ml/18fl oz per serving)

900g (2lb) chestnut mushrooms, sliced (reserve the stems for the broth)

225g (8oz) shiitake mushrooms, sliced (reserve the stems for the broth)

4 garlic cloves, chopped

1 bunch of spring onions, tops only, finely chopped (use the bulbs for the broth)

2 roasted red peppers, deseeded and chopped in to small pieces

900g (2lb) baby pak choi, thinly sliced

1.7 litres (3 pints) mushroom-soy broth (see below)

MUSHROOM-SOY BROTH

1 red onion, chopped

6 garlic cloves, roughly chopped

reserved mushroom stems

reserved spring onion bulbs

1 jalapeño chilli, halved

1 bunch of coriander (stems only)

1 tbsp olive oil

120ml (4fl oz) low-salt soy sauce

1.7 litres (3 pints) vegetable stock

To make the broth: brown the onion, garlic, mushroom stems, spring onion bulbs, chilli and coriander stems in the olive oil over medium-high heat, stirring constantly. Once the mixture is caramelised add the soy sauce and stock, and simmer for 30 minutes. Strain the broth and set aside.

To make the soup: sauté the mushrooms tops, garlic and spring onion tops until the mushrooms are tender. Pour in the broth and simmer for 20 minutes. Turn off the heat, add the roasted peppers and pak choi, cover with a lid and leave to stand for 10 minutes. Serve hot.

Nutrition: 104 calories, 2.5g fat, 12.5g carbs (4.5g sugar), 2.5g fibre, 6g protein
Exchanges: 1 protein, 3 vegetables, ½ fat

Black Bean Soup with Pico de Gallo

CLEANSE DAYS

Pico de gallo is a Mexican salsa: it adds zesty freshness to this soup. For non-Cleanse days, or for other family members, this soup tastes great with added protein.

SERVES 8 (approximately 350ml/12fl oz per serving)

450g (1lb) dried black beans, soaked overnight
1 tbsp olive oil
½ red onion, chopped
1 jalapeño chilli, sliced
½ bunch of coriander, roughly chopped
2 ripe tomatoes, chopped
1 litre (1¾ pints) vegetable stock
240ml (9fl oz) water
sea salt to taste

PICO DE GALLO
2 ripe tomatoes, deseeded and cut into small dice
½ jalapeño chilli, deseeded and finely chopped
½ bunch of coriander, finely chopped
2 tbsp finely chopped red onion
juice of 1 lemon or lime
sea salt to taste

Drain the black beans and put into a saucepan, add cold water to cover and bring to the boil for 5–10 minutes. Reduce the heat and simmer for about 1 hour or until tender. Drain excess water and set aside.

In a large saucepan, heat the olive oil and sauté onion, chilli, coriander and tomatoes for 5 minutes. Add the cooked black beans, stock and water, and simmer for 30 minutes. Transfer to a blender and blend until smooth. Season with salt to taste.

For the pico de gallo: mix the tomatoes, chilli, coriander and onion in a bowl and season with lemon or lime juice and salt to taste.

Nutrition: 220 calories, 2.5g fat, 40g carbs (10g sugar), 14g fibre, 13g protein
Exchanges: 1½ starch, 2 protein, 2 vegetables, ½ fat

❯ For additional protein, serve with grilled steak or chicken.

BURN-DAY BREAKFASTS

Oatmeal Chia Porridge BURN DAY 7

Prepare this the night before you need it for a speedy power-packed breakfast.

 30g (1oz) porridge oats
 1 tbsp chia seeds
 240ml (9fl oz) skimmed or semi-skimmed milk
 1 scoop whey protein powder
 75g (2½oz) blueberries
 1 tsp ground cinnamon

Combine the oats, chia seeds and milk in a small bowl, cover, and leave in the refrigerator overnight (at least 8 hours).

 When ready to eat, stir in the protein powder and top with blueberries and cinnamon.

Nutrition: 410 calories, 9g fat (2.5g saturated fat), 52g carbs (23g sugar), 10g fibre, 32g protein
Exchanges: 1½ starch, 1 dairy, 3 protein, 1½ fruit, 1 fat

Breakfast Oat Cookies BURN DAY 9

 30g (1oz) fine oatmeal
 ½ medium banana, mashed
 2 egg whites, lightly beaten
 2 tsp ground cinnamon
 2 tbsp chopped walnuts

Preheat the oven to 190°C/gas 5. Coat a baking sheet with cooking spray.

Put all the ingredients into a small bowl and stir until combined. Form the mixture into two cookies and place on the baking sheet. Bake for 8–10 minutes or until lightly golden. Allow to cool for 2–5 minutes then enjoy warm, or cool completely on a wire rack.

Nutrition: 310 calories, 13g fat (1.5g saturated fat), 40g carbs (8g sugar), 8g fibre, 14g protein
Exchanges: 1½ starches, 1 protein, 1 fruit, 2 fats

Peanut Butter and Egg White Porridge with Blueberries BURN DAY 13

40g (1½oz) porridge oats
120ml (4fl oz) water
3 egg whites
1 tbsp natural peanut butter
75g (2½oz) blueberries
a pinch of ground cinnamon

Mix together the oats, water and egg whites in a small heatproof bowl. Cook in the microwave on high for 2½–3 minutes. Stir in the peanut butter and top with blueberries and cinnamon.

Nutrition: 350 calories, 11g fat (2g saturated fat), 42g carbs (10g sugar), 7g fibre, 20g protein
Exchanges: 2 starches, 1½ protein, 1 fruit, 1 fat

Breakfast Tortilla + strawberries

BURN DAY 17

1 tsp rapeseed oil
75g (2½oz) red pepper, chopped
1 small onion, chopped
1 whole egg and 2 egg whites
1 wholemeal tortilla
30g (1oz) reduced-fat Cheddar cheese, grated

TO SERVE
175g (6oz) strawberries, sliced

Heat the oil in a frying pan over medium-high heat. Sauté the pepper and onion for about 8 minutes or until softened.

Meanwhile, scramble the eggs. Place the scrambled eggs on the tortilla and top with the sautéed pepper and onion and the cheese. Serve immediately, with strawberries on the side.

Nutrition: 395 calories, 15g fat (3g saturated fat), 46g carbs (13g sugar), 8g fibre, 23g protein
Exchanges: 1½ starches, 2 protein, ½ dairy, 1 fruit, 1 vegetable, 1 fat

Nut and Berry Cereal Parfait
+ hard-boiled egg BURN DAY 21

250g (9oz) fat-free plain Greek yogurt
30g (1oz) high-fibre cereal, such as Shredded Wheat
75g (2½oz) blueberries
1 tbsp chopped almonds
ground cinnamon
a pinch of stevia (optional)

TO SERVE
1 hard-boiled egg, plus 1 hard-boiled egg white

Put the yogurt in a small bowl and top with cereal, blueberries, almonds, cinnamon and stevia to taste.

Serve with a hard-boiled egg on the side.

Nutrition: 370 calories, 10g fat (2g saturated fat), 42g carbs (17g sugar), 6g fibre, 31g protein
Exchanges: 1 starch, 1+ dairy, 1 ½ protein, 1 fruit, 1 fat

BURN-DAY SNACKS (100–200 CALORIES)

- Celery sticks and 1 tbsp natural peanut butter (110 calories, 4g protein)

- 4 tbsp (60g/2oz) hummus and 100–150g (3½–5oz) raw vegetables such as cauliflower, red pepper (160 calories, 7g protein)

- 150g (5oz) grapes and 1 Babybel Light cheese or 2 Laughing Cow Light triangles (150 calories, 6g protein)

- 1 small banana and 1 tbsp natural peanut butter (180 calories, 4g protein)

- 1 small apple and 1 tbsp almond butter (160 calories, 5g protein)

- 1 small pear and 1 Babybel Light cheese or 2 Laughing Cow Light triangles (160 calories, 9g protein)

- 2 small kiwi fruit and 7 walnut halves (180 calories, 4g protein)

- 1 small orange and 1 hard-boiled egg (130 calories, 6g protein)

- ½ mango and 100-calorie pack whole almonds (150 calories, 4g protein)

- 175g (6oz) fat-free plain or vanilla Greek yogurt with 75g (2½oz) berries (130 calories, 17g protein)

BURN-DAY LUNCHES

Mexican Scramble BURN DAY 5

1 tsp coconut oil
¼ red pepper, chopped
½ small onion, chopped
60g (2oz) cooked turkey, chopped
2 tablespoons avocado, chopped
1 whole egg
2 egg whites
salt and pepper, to taste
cayenne pepper, to taste
2 small or 1 medium corn tortilla

Heat the oil in a medium frying pan over medium-high heat. Add the pepper and onion, and sauté for 4 minutes. Add the turkey and avocado, and sauté for 1 minute. Beat the egg and egg whites together. Season and stir in the cayenne. Reduce the heat to medium and add the eggs to the pan. Cook for 3 minutes, stirring often. Warm the tortillas for about 20 seconds in a small frying pan. Place the scramble in the tortillas.

Nutrition: 410 calories, 13g fat, 6g sat fat, 43g carbs, 7g fibre, 8g sugar, 30g protein
Exchanges: 1½ starches, 4 protein, 1 vegetable, 2 fats

California Turkey Wrap BURN DAY 7

60g (2oz) cooked turkey, sliced
30g (1oz) reduced-fat Cheddar cheese, sliced
1 wholemeal tortilla
2 slices avocado
85g (3oz) ripe tomatoes, chopped
about 50g (1¾oz) mixed salad leaves

TO SERVE
125g (4½oz) carrot sticks
4 tbsp fat-free plain Greek yogurt mixed with finely
    chopped dill
175g (6oz) honeydew melon, chopped

Put the turkey and cheese into the tortilla and top with avocado, tomatoes and salad leaves.

Serve with carrots and yogurt, and the melon on the side.

Nutrition: 420 calories, 11g fat (3g saturated fat), 52g carbs (16g sugar), 22g fibre, 26g protein
Exchanges: 1½ starches, 3 protein, 1+ dairy, 1 fruit, 2 vegetables, 1 fat

Tortilla Pizza with Green Salad

BURN DAY 17

1 × 20cm (8 inch) wholemeal tortilla
4 tbsp tomato sauce
1 tsp dried basil
30g (1oz) reduced-fat mozzarella, shredded
2 tbsp chopped lean cooked ham
85g (3oz) non-starchy vegetables, sliced (mushrooms,
     peppers, broccoli)

SALAD
about 100g (3½oz) romaine or other lettuce
85g (3oz) non-starchy vegetables, sliced
1 tsp olive oil
2 tsp balsamic vinegar

Preheat the oven to 180°C/gas 4. Place the tortilla on a baking sheet and top with tomato sauce, basil, cheese, ham and vegetables. Bake for 10–12 minutes. Serve with the salad.

For the salad: combine the lettuce and other vegetables in a bowl, drizzle with oil and vinegar and toss together.

Nutrition: 358 calories, 16g fat (5g saturated fat), 39g carbs (8g sugar), 9g fibre, 20g protein
Exchanges: 1½ starches, 2 protein, 3 vegetables, 1 fat

Chicken Caesar Wrap BURN DAY 9

85g (3oz) cooked chicken breast
about 50g (1¾oz) romaine lettuce, chopped
75g (2½oz) cherry tomatoes
1 wholemeal tortilla
1 tbsp grated Parmesan
1 tsp olive oil

TO SERVE
60g (2oz) carrot sticks
1 small orange

Put the chicken, lettuce and tomatoes into the tortilla. Sprinkle with Parmesan and olive oil, and wrap.

Serve with carrots, and an orange on the side.

Nutrition: 420 calories, 13g fat (3.5g saturated fat), 44g carbs (15g sugar), 9g fibre, 35g protein
Exchanges: 1½ starches, 3 protein, 1 fruit, 2½ vegetables, 1 fat

Turkey Wrap with Veggies BURN DAY 13

1 wholemeal tortilla
1 tbsp mustard
60–85g (2–3oz) turkey, sliced
30g (1oz) reduced-fat Swiss cheese, sliced
about 50g (1¾oz) mixed salad leaves
3 slices tomato

TO SERVE
175g (6oz) fat-free plain Greek yogurt
1 tbsp finely chopped fresh dill
150g (5oz) red peppers, cut into strips
115g (4oz) cucumber, cut into sticks
1 small apple

Mix together the yogurt and dill. Set aside.

Spread the tortilla with mustard. Put the turkey, cheese, salad leaves and tomato on top, and wrap.

Serve with peppers, cucumber and yogurt dip, and an apple.

Nutrition: 420 calories, 6g fat (1g saturated fat), 58g carbs (20g sugar), 10g fibre, 27g protein
Exchanges: 1½ starches, 1+ dairy, 2 protein, 1 fruit, 3 vegetables

Turkey Burger and Green Salad

BURN DAY 21

85g (3oz) lean minced turkey (venison is also a good option)
Salt and pepper
1 small (60g/2oz) wholemeal bun or thin bun
2 slices avocado

SALAD
about 100g (3½oz) romaine lettuce, young spinach leaves,
    or other salad greens
75g (2½oz) cherry tomatoes
60g (2oz) cucumber, chopped
1 tsp olive oil
2 tsp balsamic vinegar

TO SERVE
2 kiwi fruit

Season the mince and form into a burger shape. Grill the burger or cook in a frying pan or griddle pan until cooked through (when the internal temperature reaches 74°C/165°F). Place the burger on the bun and top with avocado.

For the salad: put the greens in a bowl and top with tomatoes and cucumber. Drizzle with oil and vinegar.

Serve with kiwi fruit on the side.

Nutrition: 425 calories, 14g fat (2g saturated fat), 61g carbs (23g sugar), 13g fibre, 30g protein
Exchanges: 2 starches, 3 protein, 1 fruit, 2 vegetables, 2 fat

Chicken Caprese Wrap

BURN DAY 11

A little mozzarella goes a long way in this deliciously simple lunch, and the basil adds an extra hint of Mediterranean flavour. I make filled tortillas and pittas a lot because they're tasty, satisfying and portable, so you can make them quickly at home and take them to work.

60g (2oz) cooked chicken breast
75g (2½oz) cherry tomatoes, halved
30g (1oz) mozzarella, sliced
about 50g (1¾oz) romaine lettuce, chopped
3 fresh basil leaves, finely chopped
20cm (8 inch) wholemeal tortilla
2 tsp balsamic vinegar

TO SERVE
150g (5oz) grapes

Put the chicken, tomatoes, mozzarella, lettuce and basil on the tortilla. Sprinkle over the vinegar. Serve with grapes.

Nutrition: 390 calories, 13g fat (5g saturated fat), 44g carbs (19g sugar), 6g fibre, 28g protein
Exchanges: 1½ starches, 2 protein, 1 dairy, 1 fruit, 2 vegetables

Chicken, Bean, Rice and Avocado Bowl

BURN DAY 15

85g (3oz) cooked chicken breast, sliced
85g (3oz) broccoli, chopped and steamed
75g (2½oz) canned black beans, rinsed and drained
60g (2oz) cooked brown rice
2 slices avocado
Hot sauce to taste

TO SERVE
2 kiwi fruit

Put the chicken, broccoli, beans and rice into a small bowl. Top with avocado and hot sauce.

Serve with kiwi fruit on the side.

Nutrition: 430 calories, 8g fat (1g saturated fat), 58g carbs (15g sugar), 15g fibre, 37g protein
Exchanges: 2 starches, 4 protein, 1 fruit, 1 vegetable, 1 fat

Greek Chicken and Veggie Pitta

BURN DAY 19

2 tbsp hummus
½ wholemeal pitta bread
85g (3oz) cooked chicken breast
30g (1oz) grated carrot
40g (1½oz) red pepper, chopped

TO SERVE
115g (4oz) cucumber, sliced
2 clementines

Spread the hummus into the pitta pocket, then fill with the chicken, carrot and pepper.

Serve with cucumber, and clementines on the side.

Nutrition: 340 calories, 6g fat (2g saturated fat), 49g carbs (19g sugar), 9g fibre, 28g protein
Exchanges: 1 starch, 3 protein, 1 fruit, 1½ vegetables, 1 fat

BURN-DAY DINNERS

Baked Pork Chop with Roasted Sweet Potato and Brussels Sprouts BURN DAY 7

85g (3oz) pork loin chop, fat trimmed
⅔ sweet potato, cut into small chunks
150g (5oz) Brussels sprouts, halved
1 tsp rapeseed oil

Preheat the oven to 200°C/gas 6. Place the pork chop in a small roasting pan and bake for 25–30 minutes or until cooked through (when the internal temperature reaches 63°C/145°F).

Toss the sweet potato pieces and Brussels sprouts in oil and place on a baking sheet. Bake in the oven for about 30 minutes or until the sweet potato is tender.

Nutrition: 290 calories, 10g fat (2g saturated fat), 27g carbs (7g sugar), 8g fibre, 21g protein
Exchanges: 1½ starches, 3 protein, 1½ vegetables, 1 fat

Sautéed Prawns with Broccoli + Rice
BURN DAY 11

150g (5oz) broccoli, chopped
1 tsp rapeseed oil
85–150g (3–5oz) raw prawns, peeled and deveined
2 tbsp grated Parmesan
100g (3½oz) cooked brown rice (30g/1oz raw weight)

Steam the broccoli for 5–6 minutes or until crisp-tender. Set aside.

Heat the oil in a frying pan over medium-high heat. Add the prawns and broccoli and sauté for 3–5 minutes or until the prawns are cooked through.

Sprinkle with Parmesan and serve with rice.

Nutrition: 300 calories, 10g fat (2.5g saturated fat), 29g carbs (0g sugar), 5g fibre, 25g protein
Exchanges: 1½ starches, 4 protein, ½ dairy, 1½ vegetables, 1 fat

Chicken Fajitas BURN DAY 21

1 tsp rapeseed oil
85g (3oz) chicken breast, sliced
115g (4oz) red peppers, sliced
1 small–medium onion, sliced
1 wholewheat tortilla or 2 × 15cm (6 inch) corn tortillas
4 tbsp salsa

Heat the oil in a frying pan over medium-high heat. Add the chicken and sauté for about 10 minutes.

Add the peppers and onion (spray with cooking spray, if needed) and sauté for about 10 minutes or until the vegetables are tender and the chicken is cooked through.

Put the chicken and vegetable mixture into the tortilla and top with salsa.

Nutrition: 330 calories, 10g fat (2g saturated fat), 38g carbs (9g sugar), 6g fibre, 26g protein
Exchanges: 1½ starches, 3 protein, 2½ vegetables, 1 fat

Chicken Veggie Pasta BURN DAY 19

1 tsp rapeseed oil
1 small onion, chopped
1 tsp finely chopped garlic
75g (2½oz) asparagus, cut into 2.5cm (1 inch) pieces
75g (2½oz) cherry tomatoes, halved
85g (3oz) cooked chicken, cut into bite-sized pieces
100g (3½oz) cooked wholewheat fettuccine (60g/2oz raw
    weight)
1 tsp dried oregano
1 tsp lemon juice
1 tsp grated Parmesan
Salt and pepper

Heat the oil in a large saucepan over medium-high heat. Sauté the onion and garlic for 5–10 minutes or until tender.

Meanwhile, grill or steam the asparagus.

Add the asparagus and tomatoes to the pan with the onion and garlic. Cook for about 2 minutes or until the tomatoes soften. Add the chicken, pasta, oregano, lemon juice and Parmesan and stir until well mixed. Add salt and pepper to taste and serve hot.

Nutrition: 390 calories, 9g fat (1.5g saturated fat), 43g carbs (8g sugar), 9g fibre, 36g protein
Exchanges: 1½ starches, 3 protein, 1½ vegetables, 1 fat

Prawn Stir-Fry BURN DAY 5

2 tsp rapeseed oil

350g (12oz) raw non-starchy vegetables of your choice (such
as broccoli, asparagus, mushrooms, peppers, onions),
chopped

1 tbsp low-salt soy sauce

1 tbsp water

1 tsp cornflour

¼ tsp ground ginger

¼ tsp garlic powder

85g (3oz) raw prawns, peeled and deveined

115g (4oz) cooked soba noodles (60g/2oz raw weight)

Heat the oil in a large frying pan over medium-high heat. Add
the vegetables and sauté for 8–10 minutes or until crisp-tender.

In a small bowl, mix together the soy sauce, water, cornflour,
ginger and garlic powder.

Add the prawns to the pan and sauté for 3–4 minutes or until
the prawns are cooked through.

Add the noodles and soy sauce mixture to the pan and stir-
fry for 1–2 minutes. Serve immediately.

Nutrition: 340 calories, 11g fat (2g saturated fat), 43g carbs (5g sugar),
4g fibre, 22g protein
Exchanges: 2 starches, 3 protein, 2 vegetables, 2 fats

Chicken and Vegetable Kebabs with Tzatziki + rice BURN DAY 17

85g (3oz) chicken breast, cubed

150g (5oz) red or green peppers, cut into large pieces

1 small onion, cut into wedges

75g (2½oz) cherry tomatoes

2 tsp rapeseed oil, for brushing

60g (2oz) cooked brown rice (30g/1oz raw weight), to serve

TZATZIKI

175g (6oz) fat-free plain Greek yogurt

2 tsp finely chopped garlic

1 tbsp finely chopped fresh dill

2 tsp red wine vinegar

Preheat the grill to medium-high.

Thread pieces of chicken, peppers, onion and tomatoes onto two skewers. Brush with oil. Grill for about 20 minutes, turning occasionally, until the chicken is cooked through.

For the tzatziki: in a small bowl, mix together the yogurt, garlic, dill and vinegar, and serve as a dipping sauce for the kebabs. Serve the kebabs hot, with the rice and tzatziki.

Nutrition: 450 calories, 13g fat (2g saturated fat), 36g carbs (14g sugar), 5g fibre, 48g protein

Exchanges: 1 starch, 1 dairy, 3 protein, 2 vegetables, 2 fats

Sweet and Spicy Chicken Breast with Mashed Sweet Potato and Broccoli

BURN DAY 9

1 small chicken breast, about 85g (3oz)
½ tsp dried oregano
½ tsp garlic powder
¼ tsp cayenne pepper
¼ tsp ground cumin
1 tbsp honey
½ tsp cider vinegar

BROCCOLI
150g (5oz) broccoli, chopped
1 tsp olive oil
½ tsp crushed chilli flakes
Salt and pepper

MASHED SWEET POTATO
½ small sweet potato, chopped
3 tbsp fat-free plain Greek yogurt
1 tsp garlic powder
Salt and pepper

Preheat the oven to 200°C/gas 6. Coat a baking sheet with cooking spray. Sprinkle the chicken breast with oregano, garlic, cayenne and cumin, and place on the baking sheet. Bake for 20 minutes.

Meanwhile, for the broccoli: toss the broccoli with the olive oil, chilli flakes, salt and pepper. Place on a baking sheet and bake at 200°C/gas 6 for 10–15 minutes.

For the mashed potato: boil the potato until tender, then drain. Put the potato into a bowl with the yogurt, garlic powder and salt and pepper to taste. Mash or blend with a hand mixer until smooth.

Mix the honey and vinegar together. Remove the chicken from the oven and brush or spoon half the honey mixture over the chicken. Put back in the oven and bake for about 2 minutes. Turn the chicken over, brush with the remaining honey mixture and bake for about 2 minutes or until cooked through (when the internal temperature reaches 74°C/165°F). Serve hot, with the mashed sweet potato and broccoli.

Nutrition: 350 calories, 8g fat (1.5g saturated fat), 46g carbs (27g sugar), 7g fibre, 27g protein
Exchanges: 1½ starches, 3 protein, 1½ vegetables, 1 fat

BUILD-DAY BREAKFASTS

Baked Avocado with Egg White

BUILD DAY 14

If you hard-boil a few eggs when you have 15 minutes and put them in your refrigerator, it'll save you a step when you make this and you'll have high-protein sancks ready and waiting.

½ large avocado, cut in half and stone removed
2 egg whites
Salt and pepper

TO SERVE
1 hard-boiled egg
175g (6oz) honeydew melon, chopped

Preheat the oven to 220°C/gas 7. Using a spoon, hollow out the avocado half until about 1cm (½ inch) of avocado flesh remains. Put the egg whites into the avocado and bake for about 15 minutes or until done to your liking. Season with salt and pepper. Serve with a hard-boiled egg, with melon on the side.

Nutrition: 290 calories, 16g fat (3g saturated fat), 21g carbs (16g sugar), 6g fibre, 15g protein
Exchanges: 2 protein, 1 fruit, 2+ fats

Blueberry Chia Power Protein Pudding

BUILD DAY 16

This one is super-easy but you have to prepare it the night before, so plan ahead. It'll save you time in the morning.

2 tbsp chia seeds
240ml (9fl oz) skimmed or semi-skimmed milk
1 scoop protein powder
a pinch of stevia (optional)
75g (2½oz) blueberries
1 tsp ground cinnamon

In a bowl, mix together the chia seeds, milk, protein powder and stevia to taste. Leave in the refrigerator overnight (at least 8 hours).

Top with blueberries and cinnamon, and serve.

Nutrition: 370 calories, 10g fat (2.5g saturated fat), 39g carbs (22g sugar), 11g fibre, 32g protein
Exchanges: 1 dairy, 3 protein, 1½ fruit, 2 fats

Power Protein Pancakes BUILD DAY 6

125g (4½oz) fat-free plain Greek yogurt
30g (1oz) fine oatmeal
1 whole egg
½ scoop protein powder
2 tsp ground cinnamon
75g (2½oz) blueberries

In a small bowl, stir together the yogurt, oatmeal, egg, protein powder and cinnamon until combined.

Heat a frying pan over medium-high heat. Coat the pan with cooking spray and pour in the batter to form a large pancake. Cook for 3 minutes, flip and cook for 2–3 minutes on the other side. Top with blueberries and serve.

Nutrition: 350 calories, 8g fat (2g saturated fat), 40g carbs (14g sugar), 8g fibre, 32g protein
Exchanges: 1½ starches, ½ dairy, 2½ protein, ½ fruit

Baked Egg 'Muffins' BUILD DAY 12

2 whole eggs
1 egg white
2 tbsp thinly sliced spring onions
2 tbsp chopped red pepper
2 tbsp grated reduced-fat Cheddar cheese
Salt and pepper

TO SERVE
1 small orange

Preheat the oven to 180°C/gas 4. Coat one compartment of a muffin tin with cooking spray – or use a ramekin.

Put all the ingredients into a bowl and stir until combined. Pour into the muffin tin or ramekin and bake for 10–12 minutes or until firm.

Serve hot, with an orange.

Nutrition: 260 calories, 11g fat (4g saturated fat), 19g carbs (14g sugar), 4g fibre, 21g protein
Exchanges: ½ dairy, 2½ protein, 1 fruit, ½ vegetable

Pumpkin Smoothie BUILD DAY 8

250g (9oz) canned pumpkin (no sugar added)
175g (6oz) fat-free plain yogurt
1 scoop protein powder
120ml (4fl oz) water
1 tbsp chopped walnuts
½ tsp ground cinnamon
¼ tsp each grated nutmeg and ground cloves
a pinch of stevia (optional, to taste)

Put all the ingredients into a blender and blend until smooth.

Nutrition: 340 calories, 8g fat (2g saturated fat), 40g carbs (21g sugar),
10g fibre, 23g protein
Exchanges: 1 dairy, 3 protein, 1 fruit, 1 fat

Ham and Veggie Scramble and Toast

BUILD DAY 20

1 whole egg
2 egg whites
175g (6oz) non-starchy vegetables (such as mushrooms,
    peppers, tomatoes), diced
30g (1oz) lean ham, diced
2 tbsp grated reduced-fat Cheddar cheese
1 slice of wholemeal toast
1 tbsp mashed avocado

TO SERVE
175g (6oz) honeydew melon, chopped

Beat the egg and egg whites together in a small bowl.

Heat a small frying pan over medium-high heat and coat with cooking spray. Sauté the vegetables for about 3–4 minutes or until crisp-tender. Add the ham and sauté for about 1 minute.

Pour in the eggs and cook for about 3 minutes, stirring frequently, until they are scrambled.

Add the cheese and cook for about 30 seconds or until the cheese melts. Serve at once, with avocado spreaded on the toast. Serve the melon on the side.

Nutrition: 370 calories, 11g fat (3.5g saturated fat), 36g carbs (20g sugar), 6g fibre, 32g protein
Exchanges: 1 starch, 3 protein, ½ dairy, 1 fruit, 2 vegetables, ½ fat

BUILD-DAY SNACKS (100–200 CALORIES)

- 1 Babybel Light cheese or 2 Laughing Cow Light triangles + 100-cal pack whole almonds (180 calories, 12g protein)

- 115g (4oz) low-fat cottage cheese + 75g (2½oz) cherry tomatoes (125 calories, 12g protein)

- 75g (2½oz) steamed edamame beans (100 calories, 8g protein)

- 50g (1¾oz) lean prosciutto (150 calories, 14g protein)

- 2 hard-boiled eggs (140 calories, 12g protein)

- 2 slices lean cooked ham and 1 slice reduced-fat cheese (200 calories, 16g protein)

- 175g (6oz) fat-free plain or vanilla Greek yogurt with 1 tbsp sunflower seeds (140 calories, 19g protein)

- Mini smoothie: 1 scoop vanilla protein powder + 125g (4½oz) frozen berries + 225ml (8fl oz) water (140 calories, 20g protein)

BUILD-DAY LUNCHES

Tuna Spinach Salad BUILD DAY 8

60g (2oz) fresh spinach leaves
75g (2½oz) cherry tomatoes
115g (4oz) canned tuna, drained
75g (2½oz) canned kidney beans, rinsed and drained
1 tsp olive oil
2 tsp balsamic vinegar

TO SERVE
1 small pear

Put the spinach into a bowl and top with the tomatoes, tuna and beans.

Drizzle oil and vinegar over the salad and serve, with the pear on the side.

Nutrition: 390 calories, 9g fat (1g saturated fat), 46g carbs (18g sugar), 12g fibre, 34g protein
Exchanges: 1 starch, 4 protein, 1 fruit, 1½ vegetables, 1 fat

Turkey Mushroom Scramble BUILD DAY 10

2 whole eggs
3 egg whites
Salt and pepper, to taste
1 teaspoon coconut oil
85g (3oz) chopped mushrooms (of your choice)
60g (2oz) cooked turkey, chopped
30g (1oz) spinach leaves

TO SERVE
½ plain muffin, toasted
1 teaspoon butter (optional)

Beat the eggs and egg whites together and season with salt and pepper to taste.

Heat the oil in a medium frying pan over medium-high heat. Add the mushrooms and turkey, and sauté for about 4 minutes. Add the spinach and sauté for about 1 minute, or until it has wilted.

Reduce the heat to medium. Add the eggs to pan and cook for about 3 minutes, stirring often, until you reach the desired degree of doneness.

Serve with a toasted muffin half.

Nutrition: 330 calories, 14g fat (8g saturated fat), 19g carbs, 2g fibre, 2g sugar, 35g protein
Exchanges: 4 protein, 1½ vegetables, 2 fat, 1 starch

Buffalo Chicken Salad BUILD DAY 12

115–150g (4–5oz) cooked chicken breast
1 tbsp hot sauce, such as Sriracha
about 100g (3½oz) romaine lettuce, chopped
85g (3oz) cooked quinoa
75g (2½oz) cherry tomatoes
2 tbsp crumbled blue cheese
1 tsp olive oil
2 tsp cider vinegar

TO SERVE
150g (5oz) strawberries

Toss the chicken with the hot sauce in a small bowl.

Put the lettuce in a bowl and top with the quinoa, chicken, tomatoes and blue cheese. Drizzle with oil and vinegar, and serve, with strawberries on the side.

Nutrition: 420 calories, 13g fat (3g saturated fat), 40g carbs (18g sugar), 7g fibre, 35g protein
Exchanges: 1 starch, ½ dairy, 4 protein, 1 fruit, 1 ½ vegetables, 1 fat

Chicken Bean Lettuce Wraps

BUILD DAY 14

4 butterhead or romaine lettuce leaves
150g (5oz) red peppers, sliced
115g (4oz) cooked chicken breast
75g (2½oz) cooked or canned black beans
4 tbsp salsa

TO SERVE
125g (4½oz) carrot sticks
2 tbsp hummus
75g (2½oz) cherry tomatoes
175g (6oz) cantaloupe melon, chopped

Place two lettuce leaves together on a plate, and top with half the peppers, half the chicken, half the beans and half the salsa. Repeat with the other two lettuce leaves and the remaining chicken, beans and salsa.

Serve with carrots, hummus, tomatoes and melon on the side.

Nutrition: 420 calories, 8g fat (1.5g saturated fat), 59g carbs (30g sugar), 15g fibre, 38g protein
Exchanges: 1 starch, 4 protein, 1 fruit, 3 vegetables, 1 fat

Quinoa Chicken Salad BUILD DAY 6

about 100g (3½oz) romaine lettuce, chopped
85g (3oz) cooked quinoa
115–150g (4–5oz) cooked chicken breast
75g (2½oz) red pepper, sliced
85g (3oz) cherry tomatoes
1 tsp olive oil
1 tsp balsamic vinegar

TO SERVE
1 small peach

Put the lettuce in a bowl and top with the quinoa, chicken, red pepper and tomatoes. Drizzle with oil and vinegar. Serve with a peach.

Nutrition: 410 calories, 11g fat (2g saturated fat), 36g carbs (11g sugar), 7g fibre, 42g protein
Exchanges: 1½ starch, 4 protein, 1 fruit, 2 vegetables, 1 fat

Salmon Salad Lettuce Wraps

BUILD DAY 16

85g (3oz) canned salmon
4 tbsp fat-free plain Greek yogurt
50g (1¾oz) celery, chopped
2 tbsp chopped avocado
1 tsp lemon juice
Salt and pepper
60g (2oz) cooked brown rice (30g/1oz raw weight)
4 butterhead lettuce leaves

TO SERVE
60g (2oz) baby carrots
150g (5oz) grapes

In a small bowl, mix together the salmon, yogurt, celery, avocado, lemon juice, salt and pepper.

Spoon the rice into the lettuce leaves and top with the salmon mixture. Serve with baby carrots and grapes.

Nutrition: 350 calories, 8g fat (1g saturated fat), 43g carbs (22g sugar), 6g fibre, 30g protein
Exchanges: 1 starch, 3 protein, ⅓ dairy, 1 fruit, 1½ vegetables, 1 fat

Greek Chicken Salad BUILD DAY 18

about 100g (3½oz) romaine lettuce, chopped
75g (2½oz) cherry tomatoes, halved
60g (2oz) cucumber, chopped
40g (1½oz) feta cheese, crumbled
85g (3oz) cooked chicken breast, sliced
1 tsp olive oil
1 tbsp balsamic vinegar
Salt and pepper

Put the lettuce in a bowl and top with tomatoes, cucumber, feta and chicken.

In a small bowl, mix together the oil, vinegar, salt and pepper. Pour over the salad and serve.

Nutrition: 330 calories, 16g fat (7g saturated fat), 12g carbs (8g sugar), 3g fibre, 34g protein
Exchanges: 3 protein, 1 dairy, 2 vegetables, 1 fat

Chicken 'Tacos' BUILD DAY 20

The chicken is the taco shell! This is quick, tasty and full of protein.

   115g (4oz) chicken breast
   1 tablespoon vegan mayo
   ¼ avocado, chopped
   handful of beansprouts
   Cayenne pepper, to taste
   Greek pepperoncini (mild chilli pepper), to taste

Pound the chicken breast thinly. Cook over medium heat until done through. Spread the chicken with the vegan mayo. Place all the other ingredients on the chicken and fold as a wrap.

Nutrition: 310 calories, 19g fat, 3g sat fat, 9g carbs, 4g fibre, 3g sugar, 29g protein
Exchanges: 4 protein, ½ vegetable, 2 fats

BUILD-DAY DINNERS

Fajita Salad BUILD DAY 8

1 tsp rapeseed oil
1 small onion, sliced
150g (5oz) red peppers, sliced
2 × 15cm (6 inch) corn tortillas, cut into strips
about 100g (3½oz) romaine lettuce, chopped
115–150g (4–5oz) cooked chicken breast, sliced
4 tbsp salsa

Preheat the oven to 180°C/gas 4.

Heat the oil in a frying pan over medium-high heat. Sauté the onion and peppers until tender.

Put the tortilla strips on a baking sheet and bake for about 5 minutes or until crisp and lightly golden brown.

Put the lettuce in a bowl and top with the chicken, sautéed vegetables and tortilla strips. Gently stir in the salsa.

Nutrition: 430 calories, 11g fat (2g saturated fat), 37g carbs (12g sugar), 8g fibre, 40g protein
Exchanges: 1 starch, 4 protein, 3½ vegetables, 1 fat

Portobello Beef Burger and Courgette Fries with Tomato Sauce

BUILD DAY 20

115g (4oz) lean (5% fat) minced beef

1 tsp garlic powder

Salt and pepper

2 large Portobello mushrooms, gills and stalks removed

2 slices avocado

small handful of rocket

1–2 tomato slices

COURGETTE FRIES

4 tbsp panko breadcrumbs

1 tsp dried oregano

Salt and pepper

1 courgette, cut into 7cm (3 inch) strips

1 egg white, lightly beaten

5 tbsp tomato sauce (shop-bought or homemade – see page 302), to serve

For the courgette fries: preheat the oven to 200°C/gas 6 and coat a baking sheet with cooking spray. Combine the panko, oregano, salt and pepper in a shallow dish. Dip the courgette strips into egg white and lightly dredge in the panko mixture. Place on the baking sheet and bake for 20–25 minutes or until golden brown.

For the burgers: preheat the grill over medium-high heat. Mix the beef with the garlic powder, salt and pepper, and form into a patty.

Spray the grill with cooking spray and grill the mushrooms for about 4 minutes on each side. Keep warm.

Spray the grill with a little more cooking spray and grill the beef patty for about 3 minutes on each side or until done to your liking. Place the burger on one of the mushrooms, top it with avocado, rocket, tomato and the other mushroom.

Heat the tomato sauce in the microwave or in a pan on the hob and serve with the courgettes and the burger.

Nutrition: 410 calories, 13g fat (3g saturated fat), 42g carbs (15g sugar), 9g fibre, 36g protein
Exchanges: 1 starch, 4½ protein, 4 vegetables, 1 fat

Chicken Salad with Quinoa, Cucumber and Strawberries

BUILD DAY 16

60g (2oz) fresh spinach leaves
115g (4oz) chicken breast, sliced
85g (3oz) cooked quinoa
100g (3½oz) cucumber, sliced
85g (3oz) radishes, sliced
85g (3oz) strawberries, sliced
1 tsp olive oil
2 tsp balsamic vinegar

Put the spinach in a bowl and top with the chicken, quinoa, cucumber, radishes and strawberries. Drizzle with oil and vinegar.

Nutrition: 410 calories, 12g fat (2g saturated fat), 42g carbs (18g sugar), 16g fibre, 31g protein
Exchanges: 1 starch, 4 protein, 1 fruit, 2½ vegetables, 1 fat

Salmon Cakes with Dill Sauce and Roasted Asparagus BUILD DAY 14

SALMON CAKES

115g (4oz) canned salmon, drained

4 tbsp panko breadcrumbs

2 tbsp diced red pepper

1 tbsp diced celery

2 tsp thinly sliced spring onions

1 tsp lemon juice

½ tsp finely chopped garlic

2 tbsp fat-free plain Greek yogurt

Cayenne pepper, to taste

¼ tsp each of salt and pepper

ASPARAGUS

8–10 asparagus stalks

1 tsp rapeseed oil

¼ tsp finely chopped garlic

Salt and pepper

DILL SAUCE

125g (4½oz) fat-free plain Greek yogurt

1 tbsp finely chopped dill or 2 tbsp dried dill

1 tsp lemon juice

For the salmon cakes: preheat the oven to 220°C/gas 7. Coat a baking sheet with cooking spray. Put all the ingredients into a bowl and stir until combined. Form into two patties and bake for 12–15 minutes.

For the asparagus: put the asparagus on a baking sheet and lightly toss with the oil, garlic, salt and pepper. Bake at 220°C/gas 7 for 12–15 minutes or until crisp-tender.

For the dill sauce: whisk together the yogurt, dill and lemon juice.

Serve the salmon cakes and asparagus hot, with the dill sauce.

Nutrition: 440 calories, 14g fat (2g saturated fat), 31g carbs (10g sugar), 5g fibre, 47g protein
Exchanges: 1 starch, ½ dairy, 4 protein, 3 vegetables, 1 fat

Salmon, Roasted Beetroot and Goat's Cheese Salad BUILD DAY 10

SERVES 2

2 small beetroots (or 1 large), sliced
1 tsp olive oil
230g (8oz) salmon fillet, cut into two pieces
⅛ tsp each of salt and pepper
about 150g (5oz) mixed salad leaves
60g (2oz) cucumber, sliced
60g (2oz) radishes, sliced
2 tbsp crumbled goat's cheese

DRESSING
Juice of ½ lemon
½ tsp Dijon mustard
¼ tsp finely chopped garlic
Salt and pepper
1 tsp olive oil

Preheat the oven to 200°C/gas 6. Put the beetroots on a baking sheet, toss with the olive oil and bake for 30–40 minutes, turning once.

Heat a sauté pan over medium-high heat and sprinkle the salmon with the salt and pepper. Coat the pan with cooking spray and cook the salmon for about 3–4 minutes on each side or until done to your liking.

For the dressing: stir together the lemon juice, mustard, garlic, salt and pepper. Then slowly add the olive oil, while constantly whisking.

Put the salad leaves on a plate, add the cucumber and radishes and toss with the dressing. Top with the goat's cheese, beetroot and salmon.

Nutrition (per serving): 390 calories, 16g fat (5g saturated fat), 15g carbs (7g sugar), 5g fibre, 29g protein
Exchanges (per serving): 1 starch, 4 protein, 2 vegetables, 1 fat

Turkey Meatballs and Tomato Sauce with Courgette Noodles BUILD DAY 12

115g (4oz) minced turkey breast
¼ tsp dried oregano
½ tsp finely chopped garlic
4 tbsp panko breadcrumbs
Salt and pepper

TOMATO SAUCE
1 tsp rapeseed oil
½ small onion, chopped
¼ tsp finely chopped garlic
250g (9oz) canned chopped tomatoes
Salt and pepper

COURGETTE NOODLES
2 courgettes
¼ tsp finely chopped garlic

Put the turkey, oregano, garlic, panko crumbs and some salt and pepper into a bowl and stir until well combined. Form into two or three meatballs and place in the refrigerator until ready to cook.

For the tomato sauce: heat the oil in a saucepan over medium-high heat. Sauté the onion and garlic for 5–7 minutes or until softened. Add the tomatoes, salt and pepper and reduce the heat to medium.

Put the meatballs into the sauce, cover and simmer for about 20 minutes or until the meatballs are cooked through (when the internal temperature reaches 74°C/165°F).

Meanwhile, make the courgette noodles: using a vegetable peeler, peel the courgettes into long strips. Heat a small frying pan over medium-high heat and coat with cooking spray. Add the courgettes and sauté for about 4–6 minutes or until tender. Stir in the garlic and cook for an additional 30 seconds.

Serve the meatballs and sauce over the courgette noodles.

Nutrition: 355 calories, 6g fat (1g saturated fat), 40g carbs (16g sugar), 9g fibre, 36g protein
Exchanges: 1 starch, 4 protein, 4 vegetables, 1 fat

Turkey Wraps and Salad BUILD DAY 6

115g (4oz) minced turkey breast

40g (1½oz) red pepper, finely chopped

½ small onion, finely chopped

½ tsp finely chopped garlic

¼ tsp cayenne pepper

¼ tsp each of salt and pepper

5 tbsp tomato sauce

3 tbsp water

4 butterhead or romaine lettuce leaves

2 slices avocado

4 tbsp fat-free plain Greek yogurt

SALAD

about 100g (3½oz) mixed salad leaves

40g (1½oz) cherry tomatoes

40g (1½oz) red pepper, chopped

1 tsp olive oil

1 tbsp balsamic vinegar

¼ tsp finely chopped garlic

⅛ tsp cayenne pepper

Salt and pepper

Heat a frying pan over medium-high heat. Coat with cooking spray and add the turkey, pepper, onion and garlic. Cook, stirring frequently, until the turkey is cooked and the vegetables are tender.

Add the cayenne, salt, pepper, tomato sauce and water, and simmer for about 15 minutes or until the sauce has reduced. Divide the turkey mixture among the lettuce leaves and top with avocado and yogurt.

For the salad: put the salad leaves, tomatoes and pepper into a bowl. In a small bowl, whisk together the oil, vinegar, garlic, cayenne, salt and pepper, and toss with the salad. Serve with the turkey.

Nutrition: 360 calories, 11g fat (1g saturated fat), 32g carbs (15g sugar), 10g fibre, 40g protein
Exchanges: 4 protein, 4 vegetables, 2 fats

JESSIE'S FAVOURITE FLAVOUR ENHANCERS

The recipe above is packed with flavour but if you're looking to add some to a recipe that is a little bland, here are my favourite flavour enhancers – they can really make a difference and they contain very few calories:

Apple cider vinegar

Cayenne pepper

Cinnamon

Turmeric

Fresh lemon juice

Food Exchange Options

I hope that you'll try new foods while you're on The Programme, but I have provided food category exchanges in the meal plans so that you can adjust the menus to your taste (or for other people you cook for) and still stick to the ratios for each meal or day. Use the categories below to swap foods as needed. This list is based on the American Dietetic Association Food Exchange Lists, which are available online. Where I have left the cup measurement in this is because it covers a wide range of ingredients and each one is therefore easiest to measure by volume rather than weight.

PROTEIN

Very lean protein choices have 35 calories and 1 gram of fat per serving. One serving equals:

30g (1oz) turkey breast or chicken breast, skin removed

30g (1oz) fish fillet (sole, cod, etc.)

30g (1oz) canned tuna in water

30g (1oz) shellfish (scallops, prawns etc.)

175g (6oz) cottage cheese, low-fat

2 egg whites

30g (1oz) fat-free cheese

100g (3½oz) beans, cooked (black beans, kidney, chick peas, or lentils; these count as both 1 starch and 1 very lean protein)

Lean protein choices have 55 calories and 2–3 grams of fat per serving. One serving equals:

30g (1oz) chicken (dark meat, skin removed)

30g (1oz) turkey (dark meat, skin removed)

30g (1oz) salmon, swordfish, herring

30g (1oz) lean beef (steak, tenderloin, roast beef)*

30g (1oz) veal, roast or lean chop*

30g (1oz) lamb, roast or lean chop*

30g (1oz) pork, tenderloin or fresh ham*

30g (1oz) low-fat cheese (with 3g or less of fat per ounce)

60ml (2fl oz) 4.5% cottage cheese

*Limit these choices to no more than once or twice a week. Also, when I buy meat, I try to buy organic when possible.

Medium-fat proteins have 75 calories and 5 grams of fat per serving. One serving equals:

30g (1oz) beef (any prime cut), corned beef, minced beef**

30g (1oz) pork chop

1 whole egg (medium)

30g (1oz) mozzarella cheese

60ml (2fl oz) ricotta cheese

115g (4fl oz) tofu

** Choose these very infrequently

DAIRY

Fat-free and very low-fat milk contain 90 calories per serving. One serving equals:

240ml (8½ fl oz) milk, fat-free or 1% fat

175g (6oz) yogurt, plain non-fat or low-fat

175g (6oz) plain fat-free Greek yogurt*

180ml (6 fl oz) kefir (see page 58)

30g (1oz) cheese

120ml (4fl oz) cottage cheese

Note that the composition of alternative milks made from soy, almond, rice and so on varies greatly, so if you like these, make sure the protein, carbohydrate and calcium content are meeting your needs.

* Note that cheese, cottage cheese and Greek yogurt are considered either protein or dairy. In all of the recipes they are counted as dairy to keep things simple.

FRUITS AND VEGETABLES

Fruits contain 15 grams of carbohydrate and 60 calories. One serving equals:

1 small apple, banana, orange or nectarine

1 medium peach

1 kiwi

½ grapefruit

½ mango

140g (5oz) strawberries, raspberries, or blueberries

⅛ honeydew melon

120ml (4fl oz) unsweetened juice*

*I don't recommend too much fruit juice – or dried fruit – because it's too high in sugar. Fresh is always your best option.

Vegetables contain 25 calories and 5 grams of carbohydrate. One serving equals:

½ cup (120ml) cooked vegetables (carrots, broccoli, courgette, cabbage, etc.)

1 cup (240ml) raw vegetables or salad greens

120ml (4fl oz) vegetable juice

If you are hungry while following the meal plans on The Programme, eat additional fresh or steamed vegetables! Great non-starchy vegetable choices include:

Artichokes	Cabbage (all types)
Asparagus	Carrots
Aubergine	Cauliflower
Bamboo shoots	Celery
Beans	Coleslaw, no dressing
Beansprouts	Courgette
Beetroot	Cucumber
Broccoli	Endive
Brussels sprouts	Greens (spring, etc.)

list continues ➤

Leeks

Lettuce (rocket, radicchio, romaine, chicory, endive, watercress etc.)

Mung bean sprouts

Mushrooms

Okra

Onions

Pak choi

Peppers

Sauerkraut

Spinach

Summer Squash

Swiss Chard

Tomatoes

CARBOHYDRATES

Starches/carbohydrates contain 15 grams of carbohydrate and 80 calories per serving. One serving equals:

1 slice bread (white, pumpernickel, wholemeal, rye)

¼ bagel (varies by size; one serving is 30g/1oz)

½ plain muffin

½ hamburger bun

¾ cup (180ml) dry cereal

65g rice, brown or white, cooked

50g barley or couscous, cooked

65g dried beans, peas or lentils, cooked

50g pasta, cooked

90g bulgur wheat, cooked

80g corn

75g sweet potato

80g green peas

25g popcorn, hot-air popped or microwave

FATS

Fats contain 45 calories and 5 grams of fat per serving. One serving equals:

1 teaspoon oil (coconut, walnut, vegetable, corn, rapeseed, olive, etc.)

1 teaspoon butter

1 teaspoon seeds (flaxseed, pumpkin, sunflower, sesame)

1½ teaspoons nut butter (almond, cashew, peanut; choose trans fat-free butters)

1 teaspoon mayonnaise (vegan is worth trying)

1 tablespoon salad dressing

⅛ avocado (about 30g/1oz)

8 large black olives

1 slice nitrate-free bacon

2 tablespoons grated coconut

Index

Acknowledgements

Thank you to my mother, Terri, for teaching me what love and compassion are, and to my father, Mike, one of the hardest working men I know, who still finds time to chase his dreams. Thank you to my son, Rowan: I had forgotten how important it is to appreciate every minute until you came into my life. I am continually inspired by the experiences and courage of the amazing people I have trained, and I am grateful for everything they teach me, especially about how important it is to listen and to believe in yourself. A special thanks to Stacy Creamer at Hachette Books, for believing in me and what I do; to Melissa Moore, one rad writer; and to Dr Melina Jampolis, Ashley Marriott, and my team Jill Tipping, Ryan Haden, Scott Howard and Richard Abate for their help with The Programme.